T0249790

Geriatric Otolaryngology

Editors

NATASHA MIRZA
JENNIFER Y. LEE

OTOLARYNGOLOGIC CLINICS OF NORTH AMERICA

www.oto.theclinics.com

Consulting Editor
SUJANA S. CHANDRASEKHAR

August 2018 • Volume 51 • Number 4

ELSEVIER

1600 John F. Kennedy Boulevard • Suite 1800 • Philadelphia, Pennsylvania, 19103-2899

http://www.oto.theclinics.com

OTOLARYNGOLOGIC CLINICS OF NORTH AMERICA Volume 51, Number 4
August 2018 ISSN 0030-6665, ISBN-13: 978-0-323-61406-1

Editor: Jessica McCool
Developmental Editor: Sara Watkins

© **2018 Elsevier Inc. All rights reserved.**

This periodical and the individual contributions contained in it are protected under copyright by Elsevier, and the following terms and conditions apply to their use:

Photocopying

Single photocopies of single articles may be made for personal use as allowed by national copyright laws. Permission of the Publisher and payment of a fee is required for all other photocopying, including multiple or systematic copying, copying for advertising or promotional purposes, resale, and all forms of document delivery. Special rates are available for educational institutions that wish to make photocopies for non-profit educational classroom use. For information on how to seek permission visit www.elsevier.com/permissions or call: (+44) 1865 843830 (UK)/(+1) 215 239 3804 (USA).

Derivative Works

Subscribers may reproduce tables of contents or prepare lists of articles including abstracts for internal circulation within their institutions. Permission of the Publisher is required for resale or distribution outside the institution. Permission of the Publisher is required for all other derivative works, including compilations and translations (please consult www.elsevier.com/permissions).

Electronic Storage or Usage

Permission of the Publisher is required to store or use electronically any material contained in this periodical, including any article or part of an article (please consult www.elsevier.com/permissions). Except as outlined above, no part of this publication may be reproduced, stored in a retrieval system or transmitted in any form or by any means, electronic, mechanical, photocopying, recording or otherwise, without prior written permission of the Publisher.

Notice

No responsibility is assumed by the Publisher for any injury and/or damage to persons or property as a matter of products liability, negligence or otherwise, or from any use or operation of any methods, products, instructions or ideas contained in the material herein. Because of rapid advances in the medical sciences, in particular, independent verification of diagnoses and drug dosages should be made.

Although all advertising material is expected to conform to ethical (medical) standards, inclusion in this publication does not constitute a guarantee or endorsement of the quality or value of such product or of the claims made of it by its manufacturer.

Otolaryngologic Clinics of North America (ISSN 0030-6665) is published bimonthly by Elsevier, Inc., 360 Park Avenue South, New York, NY 10010-1710. Months of issue are February, April, June, August, October, and December. Business and Editorial Offices: 1600 John F. Kennedy Blvd., Suite 1800, Philadelphia, PA 19103-2899. Customer Service Office: 6277 Sea Harbor Drive, Orlando, FL 32887-4800. Periodicals postage paid at New York, NY and additional mailing offices. Subscription prices are $396.00 per year (US individuals), $835.00 per year (US institutions), $100.00 per year (US student/resident), $519.00 per year (Canadian individuals), $1058.00 per year (Canadian institutions), $556.00 per year (international individuals), $1058.00 per year (international institutions), $270.00 per year (international & Canadian student/resident). Foreign air speed delivery is included in all *Clinics*' subscription prices. All prices are subject to change without notice. **POSTMASTER:** Send address changes to *Otolaryngologic Clinics of North America,* Elsevier Health Sciences Division, Subscription Customer Service, 3251 Riverport Lane, Maryland Heights, MO 63043. **Telephone: 1-800-654-2452 (U.S. and Canada); 314-447-8871 (outside U.S. and Canada). Fax: 314-447-8029. E-mail: journalscustomerservice-usa@elsevier.com (for print support); journalsonlinesupport-usa@elsevier.com (for online support).**

Reprints. For copies of 100 or more of articles in this publication, please contact the Commercial Reprints Department, Elsevier Inc., 360 Park Avenue South, New York, NY 10010-1710. Tel.: 212-633-3874; Fax: 212-633-3820; E-mail: reprints@elsevier.com.

Otolaryngologic Clinics of North America is also published in Spanish by McGraw-Hill Interamericana Editores S.A., P.O. Box 5-237, 06500 Mexico D.F., Mexico.

Otolaryngologic Clinics of North America is covered in *MEDLINE/PubMed (Index Medicus), Current Contents/Clinical Medicine, Excerpta Medica, BIOSIS, Science Citation Index,* and *ISI/BIOMED.*

PROGRAM OBJECTIVE

The goal of the *Otolaryngologic Clinics of North America* is to provide information on the latest trends in patient management, the newest advances; and provide a sound basis for choosing treatment options in the field of otolaryngology.

LEARNING OBJECTIVES

Upon completion of this activity, participants will be able to:

1. Review Age Related Hearing Loss and Deficits in Taste and Smell.
2. Discuss Endocrine Surgery and Facial Plastic Surgery in the Geriatric Population, as well as, Opportunities and Challenges for Otolaryngology-Head and Neck Surgery.
3. Recognize the Effects of Reflux, Voice Changes, and Dysphagia in the Elderly Patient.

ACCREDITATION

The Elsevier Office of Continuing Medical Education (EOCME) is accredited by the Accreditation Council for Continuing Medical Education (ACCME) to provide continuing medical education for physicians.

The EOCME designates this enduring material for a maximum of 15 *AMA PRA Category 1 Credit*(s)™. Physicians should claim only the credit commensurate with the extent of their participation in the activity.

All other health care professionals requesting continuing education credit for this enduring material will be issued a certificate of participation.

DISCLOSURE OF CONFLICTS OF INTEREST

The EOCME assesses conflict of interest with its instructors, faculty, planners, and other individuals who are in a position to control the content of CME activities. All relevant conflicts of interest that are identified are thoroughly vetted by EOCME for fair balance, scientific objectivity, and patient care recommendations. EOCME is committed to providing its learners with CME activities that promote improvements or quality in healthcare and not a specific proprietary business or a commercial interest.

The planning committee, staff, authors and editors listed below have identified no financial relationships or relationships to products or devices they or their spouse/life partner have with commercial interest related to the content of this CME activity:

Jennifer C. Alyono, MD, MS; Arnaud F. Bewley, MD; Eric W. Cerrati, MD; Brian P. Cervenka, MD; Brandon L. Chiu, MD; Audrey Chun, MD; David Eibling, MD; Nazaneen Grant, MD; Kristen Helm; David W. Hsu, MD; Alison Kemp; Karen Kost, MD; Jiahui Lin, MD; Susan McCammon, MD, FACS; Jessica McCool; John Benjamin McIntire, MD; Jayme Meiner, MS; Abie H. Mendelsohn, MD; Eric R. Mong, BS; Samia Nawaz, MS; Ian Newberry, MD; Jayant M. Pinto, MD, FACS; Shyam Rao, MD; Sarah K. Rapoport, MD; Jeffrey D. Suh, MD; Maria Suurna, MD, FACS; J. Regan Thomas, MD; Ozlem E. Tulunay-Ugur, MD; Yona Vaisbuch, MD.

The planning committee, staff, authors and editors listed below have identified financial relationships or relationships to products or devices they or their spouse/life partner have with commercial interest related to the content of this CME activity:

Richard L. Doty, PhD, FAAN: receives royalties and/or holds a patent with Cambridge University Press, Johns Hopkins University Press, and John Wiley & Sons, Inc. Dr. Doty also has acted as a consultant/advisor for Johnson & Johnson Services, Inc. and Merck & Co., Inc. and owns stock in Sensonics.

Jennifer Y. Lee, MD: Jennifer.Y.Lee@stanford.edu
Natasha Mirza, MD, FACS: Natasha.Mirza@uphs.upenn.edu
Peter Luke Santa Maria, MD, PhD: is a consultant/advisor for EarLens Corporation

UNAPPROVED/OFF-LABEL USE DISCLOSURE

The EOCME requires CME faculty to disclose to the participants:

1. When products or procedures being discussed are off-label, unlabelled, experimental, and/or investigational (not US Food and Drug Administration [FDA] approved); and
2. Any limitations on the information presented, such as data that are preliminary or that represent ongoing research, interim analyses, and/or unsupported opinions. Faculty may discuss information about pharmaceutical agents that is outside of FDA-approved labelling. This information is intended solely for CME and is not intended to promote off-label use of these medications. If you have any questions, contact the medical affairs department of the manufacturer for the most recent prescribing information.

TO ENROLL

To enroll in the *Otolaryngologic Clinics of North America* Continuing Medical Education program, call customer service at 1-800-654-2452 or sign up online at http://www.theclinics.com/home/cme. The CME program is available to subscribers for an additional annual fee of USD 260.

METHOD OF PARTICIPATION

In order to claim credit, participants must complete the following:

1. Complete enrolment as indicated above.
2. Read the activity.
3. Complete the CME Test and Evaluation. Participants must achieve a score of 70% on the test. All CME Tests and Evaluations must be completed online.

CME INQUIRIES/SPECIAL NEEDS

For all CME inquiries or special needs, please contact elsevierCME@elsevier.com.

Contributors

CONSULTING EDITOR

SUJANA S. CHANDRASEKHAR, MD
Past President, American Academy of Otolaryngology-Head and Neck Surgery, Partner, ENT & Allergy Associates, LLP, Clinical Professor, Department of Otolaryngology–Head and Neck Surgery, Zucker School of Medicine at Hofstra-Northwell, Hempstead, New York, USA; Clinical Associate Professor, Department of Otolaryngology–Head and Neck Surgery, Icahn School of Medicine at Mount Sinai, New York, New York, USA

EDITORS

NATASHA MIRZA, MD, FACS
Professor, Otolaryngology–Head and Neck Surgery, University of Pennsylvania, Director, Penn Center for Voice and Swallowing, Chief of Otolaryngology, Philadelphia VA Medical Center, Hospital of the University of Pennsylvania, Philadelphia, Pennsylvania, USA

JENNIFER Y. LEE, MD
Assistant Professor, Otolaryngology–Head and Neck Surgery, Stanford University, Division Chief of Comprehensive Otolaryngology, Clinic Chief of Adult Otolaryngology, Palo Alto, California, USA

AUTHORS

JENNIFER C. ALYONO, MD, MS
Department of Otolaryngology–Head and Neck Surgery, Stanford University, Stanford, California, USA

ARNAUD F. BEWLEY, MD
Department of Otolaryngology, Division of Head and Neck Surgery, University of California, Davis, Sacramento, California, USA

ERIC W. CERRATI, MD
Facial Plastic and Reconstructive Surgery, Division of Otolaryngology–Head and Neck Surgery, University of Utah, Salt Lake City, Utah, USA

BRIAN P. CERVENKA, MD
Department of Otolaryngology, Division of Head and Neck Surgery, University of California, Davis, Sacramento, California, USA

BRANDON L. CHIU, MD
Section of Otolaryngology–Head and Neck Surgery, The University of Chicago, Chicago, Illinois, USA

AUDREY CHUN, MD
Associate Professor, Department of Geriatrics and Palliative Medicine, Icahn School of Medicine at Mount Sinai, New York, New York, USA

RICHARD L. DOTY, PhD, FAAN
Professor and Director, Smell and Taste Center, Department of Otorhinolaryngology, Head and Neck Surgery, Perelman School of Medicine, University of Pennsylvania, Philadelphia, Pennsylvania, USA

DAVID EIBLING, MD
Professor, Department of Otolaryngology–Head and Neck Surgery, University of Pittsburgh School of Medicine, Pittsburgh, Pennsylvania, USA

NAZANEEN GRANT, MD
Associate Professor of Otolaryngology–Head and Neck Surgery, MedStar Georgetown University Hospital, Washington, DC, USA

DAVID W. HSU, MD
Rhinology Fellow and Clinical Instructor, Department of Head and Neck Surgery, UCLA, Los Angeles, California, USA

KAREN KOST, MD
Professor, Department of Otolaryngology–Head and Neck Surgery, McGill University School of Medicine, Montreal, Québec, Canada

JIAHUI LIN, MD
Department of Otolaryngology–Head and Neck Surgery, NewYork-Presbyterian Hospital, Columbia and Weill Cornell, New York, New York, USA

SUSAN McCAMMON, MD, FACS
Department of Otolaryngology, The University of Texas Medical Branch at Galveston, Galveston, Texas, USA

JOHN BENJAMIN McINTIRE, MD
Department of Otolaryngology, The University of Texas Medical Branch at Galveston, Galveston, Texas, USA

JAYME MEINER, MS
Department of Physical Medicine and Rehabilitation, MedStar Georgetown University Hospital, Washington, DC, USA

ABIE H. MENDELSOHN, MD
Assistant Professor-in-Residence, Department of Head and Neck Surgery, UCLA Voice Center for Medicine and the Arts, David Geffen School of Medicine at UCLA, Los Angeles, California, USA

ERIC R. MONG, BS
The University of Texas Medical Branch at Galveston, Galveston, Texas, USA

SAMIA NAWAZ, MS
Department of Otolaryngology–Head and Neck Surgery, University of Arkansas for Medical Sciences, Little Rock, Arkansas, USA

IAN NEWBERRY, MD
Facial Plastic and Reconstructive Surgery, Division of Otolaryngology–Head and Neck Surgery, University of Utah, Salt Lake City, Utah, USA

JAYANT M. PINTO, MD, FACS
Center on Demography and Economics of Aging, The University of Chicago, Chicago, Illinois, USA

SHYAM RAO, MD
Department of Radiation Oncology, University of California, Davis, Sacramento, California, USA

SARAH K. RAPOPORT, MD
Department of Otolaryngology–Head and Neck Surgery, MedStar Georgetown University Hospital, Washington, DC, USA

PETER LUKE SANTA MARIA, MD, PhD
Assistant Professor, Neurotology Division, Otolaryngology–Head and Neck Surgery, Stanford University, Stanford, California, USA

JEFFREY D. SUH, MD
Associate Professor, Department of Head and Neck Surgery, UCLA, Los Angeles, California, USA

MARIA SUURNA, MD, FACS
Assistant Professor, Department of Otolaryngology–Head and Neck Surgery, Weill Cornell Medicine, NewYork-Presbyterian Hospital, New York, New York, USA

J. REGAN THOMAS, MD
Division of Facial Plastic and Reconstructive Surgery, Department of Otolaryngology–Head and Neck Surgery, Northwestern University, Chicago, Illinois, USA

OZLEM E. TULUNAY-UGUR, MD
Associate Professor, Director, Division of Laryngology, Department of Otolaryngology–Head and Neck Surgery, University of Arkansas for Medical Sciences, Little Rock, Arkansas, USA

YONA VAISBUCH, MD
Clinical Instructor, Neurotology Division, Otolaryngology–Head and Neck Surgery Department, Stanford University, Stanford, California, USA

Contents

The number of Americans over the age of 65 years has been growing much faster than the overall population's growth rate. This change can be largely attributed to the improvement in life expectancy. This demographic shift yields a unique and exciting opportunity to provide both expedient and cost-efficient care to a growing patient population.

Age-related hearing loss is a multifactorial condition that affects more than one-third of the aging population. Left untreated it can increase the risk of cognitive decline, dementia, social isolation, depression, and falls. Hearing augmentation devices exhibit improved digital sound processing and smartphone connectivity. Stigma remains one of the prominent barriers, and devices available at present offer in the canal models, miniature sizes, and camouflage with the hair or skin color. Although rigorous scientific research of inner ear regeneration is ongoing and some clinical early-phase studies do exist, the clinical availability is still some time away.

Vertigo and dizziness are common conditions among older adults. They are closely associated with fall risk and portend major implications for geriatric injury and disability. Management can be particularly challenging, because symptoms are often nonspecific and may reflect multiple causes. Chronic dizziness can reflect dysfunction in the vestibular, somatosensory, or visual systems or in their central integration. Systemic processes, such as postural hypotension, arrhythmias, heart failure, medication use, and lower extremity weakness or frailty, also contribute. Management of acute vestibular syndrome requires ruling out dangerous causes, such as stroke. This article reviews relevant definitions, epidemiology, pathophysiology, diagnosis, and clinical management.

Management of head and neck cancer in the elderly patient is particularly challenging given the high morbidity associated with treatment. Surgery, radiotherapy, and chemotherapy have all been demonstrated as effective in older patients; however, older patients are more susceptible to treatment-induced toxicity, which can limit the survival benefits of certain interventions. This susceptibility is better associated with the presence of multiple comorbidities and decreasing functional status than with age alone. Screening tools allow for risk stratification, treatment deintensification, and even treatment avoidance in patients who are deemed to be at high risk of being harmed by standard therapy.

Age must be a factor when considering endocrine surgery. Age itself is a risk factor for complications after thyroidectomy, specifically pulmonary, infectious, and cardiac complications. For this reason, in patients with nodular thyroid disease or thyroid microcarcinoma, length of observation must be measured against age and surgical risk. Outcomes of thyroid surgery in geriatric patients can be improved with several measures, including careful preoperative risk stratification based on comorbidities and frailty. In this population subset, it is imperative to have an earnest discussion with patients, their families, and any surrogate decision maker regarding potential outcomes of treatment versus observation.

The impact of aging is as inevitable in the larynx as on all biologic systems. The muscles of the larynx have the potential to atrophy, the elastin fibers of lamina propria thin with age, and mucous production diminishes. As a result, vocal folds fail to approximate appropriately and the stress on once-robust vocal folds increases. These changes present as poor voice quality, vocal tension, tremor, and altered fundamental frequency. Rather than consider presbyphonia as an immutable diagnosis, one must see it as an opportunity to elevate the standard of care and set goals to work for therapeutic improvement of voice quality.

Dysphagia in older adults is a challenging problem and necessitates a team approach. The key to effective management is recognition. Patients tend to dismiss their symptoms as normal aging; therefore, early diagnosis depends on the diligence of the primary care doctors. No diagnostic technique can replace the benefits of a thorough history, with a detailed understanding of nutritional status and aspiration risk. Although one of the main goals in management is to ensure safe swallowing, the impact of a nonoral diet on the quality of life of patients should not be underestimated.

Reflux-related complaints are a frequent cause for otolaryngology consultation, and with the aging population the concerns specific to the elderly patient with reflux are critical. The elderly patient is less likely to present with typical laryngopharyngeal reflux (LPR) or gastroesophageal reflux disease (GERD) symptoms. Elderly patients typically have objective findings more severe than the level of the symptoms. Therefore, upfront invasive esophageal testing as opposed to an initial medical therapy trial is the recommended management strategy. For all patients irrespective of age, lifestyle and diet modifications continue to represent the cornerstone of medical management for LPR and GERD.

Greater life expectancy with advancements in technology and medicine has led to an increasing interest in facial rejuvenation. Facial aging is an inevitable process that largely results from soft tissue descent and volumetric deflation. However, a comprehensive knowledge of the aging process and precise assessment of the exact pathologies yielding the patient's senescent appearance is essential to produce the best cosmetic outcome. The surgeon must evaluate each region independently and the aging face as a whole to ensure a pleasing, natural appearance.

Rhinitis and sinusitis are common medical conditions that affect the geriatric population and have a significant impact on the quality of life. Because few studies examine differences in the clinical management between the geriatric and general adult population, therapies should be based on current guidelines. Special considerations should be made when treating these patients in regards to multiple comorbidities and the potential for drug interactions from polypharmacy. Further research on the pathogenesis of sinusitis in the geriatric population may provide specific differences in the clinical management in this population.

Disturbances in both the ability to smell and to taste are common in older persons. Such disturbances influence nutrition, safety, quality of life, and psychological and physical health. The anatomic and physiologic causes of age-related disturbances are multiple and interacting and depend on genetic and environmental factors. Frank losses of function, distortions, and hallucinations are common. Most distortions resolve over time, although this can take months or even years. Olfactory dysfunction occurs during the earliest stages of several neurologic disorders, most notably Alzheimer disease and Parkinson disease, likely heralding the onset of the underlying pathologies.

OTOLARYNGOLOGIC CLINICS
OF NORTH AMERICA

ISSUE OF RELATED INTEREST

Clinics in Geriatric Medicine, May 2018 (Vol. 34, No. 2)
Geriatric Otolaryngology
Karen M. Kost, *Editor*
Available at: http://www.geriatric.theclinics.com/

THE CLINICS ARE AVAILABLE ONLINE!
Access your subscription at:
www.theclinics.com

Foreword

Treating the Elderly with Science and Dignity

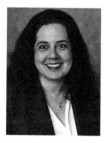

Sujana S. Chandrasekhar, MD
Consulting Editor

Just as children are not simply small adults, elderly individuals have medical needs that may not be satisfied by just translating medical knowledge from younger adults. Geriatric medicine deals exclusively with the health and diseases of the elderly, including many issues that affect them primarily due to the aging of organs over time, such as cataracts, dementia, and presbycusis, among others. A challenge in this population is that care of one problem must include consideration of a multitude of parameters, including coexistent illnesses and polypharmacy, for better decision making.

The term "geriatrics" was coined in 1909, when only 4% of the US population was over age 65, and the average life expectancy in this country was only 45 years. Access to health care was expanded in 1965 by the creation of Medicare and Medicaid and passage of the Older Americans Act. Separate Geriatrics Departments were established in US Medical Schools starting in 1982. As more patients have been cared for in a rigorous and scientific fashion, our knowledge has expanded. Fifteen percent of the US population in 2015 was over age 65, and that number will be 22% by 2050. Current US life expectancy is 79 years. Expectations for good or great quality of life are high in these patients and their families.

Drs Natasha Mirza and Jennifer Lee have spearheaded a thorough compilation of expert articles touching all facets of Geriatric Otolaryngology in this issue of *Otolaryngologic Clinics of North America*. Presbycusis is managed at a much higher level now than it was before, with earlier diagnosis and vast improvements in amplification and hearing augmentation over the squealing, crackly analog devices of yesteryear. Telling a dizzy elderly person that they are just old and they should not walk is denying them the evaluation and care that is available to them. Dr Alyono masterfully bridges the gap between inner ear disorders and the significant risk and consequences of falls in the elderly. As we expect our patients to live longer, treatment of head and neck cancer in these patients, once relegated to palliation, is now tailored for cure. Along with

Otolaryngol Clin N Am 51 (2018) xv–xvi
https://doi.org/10.1016/j.otc.2018.04.003
0030-6665/18/© 2018 Published by Elsevier Inc.

the advances in endocrine surgery in general comes the particular care needed when caring for thyroid and parathyroid problems in the over-65 age group. This is detailed by Drs McIntire, McCammon, and Mong.

Communication problems in the elderly are not by any means limited to hearing loss. Changes in voice may make conversations challenging. Swallowing concerns may limit their participation in the societal rituals of eating meals with others. Both underlying disease and use of multiple medications may cause reflux that can further impair speech and swallow. The articles on these subjects stand alone comfortably but read together form a thorough primer on these issues in the elderly.

When the average life expectancy is nearly 80, and many individuals are living to 90 and 100, it is not unreasonable to expect that elderly patients would want cosmetic surgery to diminish the visible effects of aging. Drs Newberry, Cerrati, and Thomas review the special concerns of counseling on, and performing, facial plastic surgery in the over-65s. Upper airway issues may occur concomitantly or separately. There are particular issues regarding rhinitis in the elderly that have to do with aging mucosa. These can affect quality of life in and of themselves but can also predispose to sinusitis and age-related deficits in smell and taste. Comfortable sleep is often elusive in the older population; again, like imbalance, this does not have to be "accepted" and should be evaluated and treated. The articles on these subjects are very informative, and I recommend them highly.

When contemplating any surgery on any patient, we as surgeons need to know what types of evaluations are needed to optimize that patient's care. The elderly may have multiple medical problems, be on many medications, and need particular help in terms of food and social support. As the field of Geriatric Otolaryngology develops, our colleagues can help both otolaryngologists and geriatricians understand the intersection of the fields, which results in improved care for all patients.

Again, I commend Drs Mirza and Lee and all of the authors on their strong work in bringing this excellent issue of *Otolaryngologic Clinics of North America* on Geriatric Otolaryngology to you, the reader. I hope that you enjoy it and find it to be helpful in your practice.

Sujana S. Chandrasekhar, MD
ENT & Allergy Associates, LLP
18 East 48th Street, 2nd Floor
New York, NY 10017, USA

E-mail address:
ssc@nyotology.com

Preface

Geriatric Otolaryngology

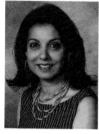 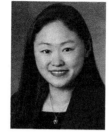

Natasha Mirza, MD, FACS   Jennifer Y. Lee, MD
Editors

According to the US census publications, the US population is expected to grow by 27% between 2012 and 2050, which would be an increase from 314 million to 400 million. About 80 million in the US are expected to be over 65 years old. The projection of increased elderly population is due to several factors: increase in life expectancy, decrease in mortality, and decrease in fertility. As such, the recognition of the geriatric patient with otolaryngologic problems will present some unique challenges. This is however also an opportunity to provide improved and specialty-specific management to these individuals in a safe and cost-efficient manner.

This issue of the *Otolaryngology Clinics of North America* is dedicated to the understanding of the emerging field of Geriatric Otolaryngology. It is timely to recognize that the aging population has somewhat different pathologies, presentations, and management challenges. The authors were chosen because of their expertise and national reputation, and we are deeply indebted for their time and effort in writing these articles and enhancing our knowledge in this field. A diverse group of topics are covered that should be of interest to all who take care of patients in this age group.

The authors have provided an in-depth review of the economics of the aging population, along with a most interesting history of this emerging subspecialty. They have addressed the needs of "baby boomers" and have comprehensively suggested ways to keep pace with this increase in health care demand. Decrements and alterations in sensory functions such as hearing, balance, smell, and taste are covered, along with a discussion on the significant impact these subtle changes can have in the day-to-day life of the elderly. The medical and preoperative evaluation of geriatric patients and the general practice guidelines that help stratify the elderly preoperative patient concentrating on cardiac and pulmonary risk evaluations are elucidated and provide helpful guidelines for the practicing otolaryngologist on the preoperative discussions.

Otolaryngol Clin N Am 51 (2018) xvii–xviii
https://doi.org/10.1016/j.otc.2018.04.002
0030-6665/18/© 2018 Published by Elsevier Inc.

Voice alterations and swallowing dysfunction affect communication ability and the ability of an elderly individual to maintain their health. In fact, vague symptoms of dysphagia may be related to frailty or even laryngopharyngeal reflux. Management with medications, and more importantly with lifestyle and diet modifications, is discussed. The importance of recognizing which patients with endocrine disorders are better off being observed rather than undergoing the risks of surgery is described. Some of the most common adult health-related problems in the United States pertain to sinusitis and obstructive sleep apnea. Both conditions significantly affect the geriatric population, and surgical and nonsurgical management strategies are considered along with special consideration to the comorbidities.

Our authors have delved into the complexities of managing patients with head and neck cancer with the high morbidity associated with treatment. The literature supports treatment, whether surgery, radiotherapy, and/or chemotherapy, to be as effective in the elderly; however, as this population is more susceptible to the side effects and toxicity of treatment, methods to decrease issues and consideration of weighing the risks and benefits of each treatment are very nicely laid out.

Attempts to gracefully age and enhance the appearance of elderly individuals are addressed along with ways that allow practitioners to better understand the appropriate candidates and how best to achieve their goal of facial rejuvenation.

Our hope is that this issue of *Otolaryngology Clinics of North America* will provide the practicing otolaryngologist, who will inevitably be taking care of an increasing number of geriatric patients, with a reference guide to approach specific issues in a more knowledgeable and comprehensive manner and tailor care accordingly. We hope that you find these discussions useful to your practice.

Natasha Mirza, MD, FACS
Otolaryngology, Head and Neck Surgery
University of Pennsylvania
Penn Voice and Swallowing Center
Philadelphia VA Medical Center
5 Silverstein
3400 Spruce Street
Philadelphia, PA 19010, USA

Jennifer Y. Lee, MD
Otolaryngology, Head and Neck Surgery
Stanford University
Comprehensive Otolaryngology
Adult Otolaryngology
801 Welch Road, Second Floor
Palo Alto, CA 94305, USA

E-mail addresses:
Natasha.Mirza@uphs.upenn.edu (N. Mirza)
Jennifer.Y.Lee@stanford.edu (J.Y. Lee)

Aging in the United States
Opportunities and Challenges for
Otolaryngology–Head and Neck Surgery

Brandon L. Chiu, MD[a], Jayant M. Pinto, MD[b],*

KEYWORDS

- Demographic shift yield • Growing patient population • Baby boomer generation
- Congressional Budget Office • Geriatric Otolaryngology • Otolaryngology Workforce

KEY POINTS

- The number and percentage of Americans over the age of 65 years are increasing.
- These changes can be largely attributed to the improvement in life expectancy.
- This demographic shift will cause an increased demand for care in otolaryngology, which will have to be met by changes to clinical practice, workforce adjustment, and/or a combination of both.

DEMOGRAPHIC TRENDS

Over the past decade, the demographic profile of the United States has been evolving at an increasing rate. From 2005 to 2015, the number of Americans over the age of 65 years, defined as the population of older adults, increased by over 12 million people, from 35 million to 47 million according to the US Census Bureau.[1] This segment has been growing much faster than the overall population's growth rate; older adults represent more than 14% of the population, which is up from 12% during that same time period. Similar trends are present in other developed nations. Worldwide, the population of older adults has increased from 524 million in 2010 (7.6%) to 608 million in 2015 (8.3%).[2]

These changes can be largely attributed to the improvement in life expectancy. Life expectancy was 62 years in the 1980s and now exceeds 70 years worldwide.[2] In the United States, life expectancy increased from 74 years to over 78 years. Although many factors are responsible for this benefit, advances in health care are some of

Disclosure: The authors have nothing to disclose.
[a] Section of Otolaryngology–Head and Neck Surgery, The University of Chicago, 5841 S Maryland Avenue, Chicago, IL 60637, USA; [b] Center on Demography and Economics of Aging, The University of Chicago, MC1035, Room E103, 5841 South Maryland Avenue, Chicago, IL 60637, USA
* Corresponding author.
E-mail address: jpinto@surgery.bsd.uchicago.edu

the main drivers of this change. Examples of such improvements, among many, include changes in health behaviors like smoking cessation and decreased alcohol consumption, new technology and imaging modalities making earlier diagnoses possible, and exponential growth in the development of prescription medications. Although the increase in life expectancy in the United States is less than the world as a whole, it is anticipated that the US population will continue to grow older over the next few decades. The aging of the baby boomer generation (individuals born after World War II in the mid-1940s to the early 1960s) is driving the first wave of this accelerated demographic shift. They started entering retirement age and can be expected to further increase the population of older adults by an annualized rate of 3% through 2030. As a result, there will be an estimated 74 million older adults in the United States in 2030 and these people will comprise approximately 20% of the total population at that time.[3] The purpose of this article is to raise awareness of this evolving population change among otolaryngologists, so that they can adapt practices and prepare to care for the nation's older patients.

ECONOMICS OF HEALTH CARE FOR THE POPULATION OF OLDER ADULTS

With this clear shift toward an aging United States, there will come a concomitant change in the demands for medical and surgical services. Even prior to the influx of the baby boomers, older adults accounted for 26% of all physician office visits and 35% of all hospital stays.[4] These figures will continue to rise. This current increase in demand has garnered much attention and has been an area of significant concern among clinicians, policy makers, health administrators, and politicians. In fact, the Congressional Budget Office has already budgeted the cost of Medicare to double over the next decade, with payments going from $692 billion in 2016 to an estimated $1402 billion in 2027.[5]

Aging of the US population has been occurring for some time. Even in 2002, considerable shortages in geriatricians were anticipated by the Alliance for Aging Research. At that time, there was already a shortage of 12,000 doctors, with projected deficits in the number of needed clinicians to increase to 28,000 by 2030. More recently, the Association of American Medical Colleges released a report in 2017 stating continued shortfalls in physician supply in response in this growing demand. With a total of approximately 800,000 physicians in the United States as of 2015, the projected shortfall by 2030 is expected to be between 40,800 and 104,900 practitioners.[6] These numbers have improved slightly compared with previous years' projections due to a focus on primary care, with increased supply of nurse practitioners and other physician extenders, in addition to other federal government initiatives. Furthermore, other health care services have also responded to this increase in demand. According to the Bureau of Labor Statistics, 13 of the top 20 fastest growing occupations in the United States in 2015 are health care related: home health aides, physician assistants, and physical therapists.[7] The supply of surgical subspecialists, however, is not expected to change substantially, with shortfalls between 19,800 and 29,000 surgeons expected by 2030.[6]

THE LANDSCAPE OF THE OTOLARYNGOLOGY WORKFORCE

Data from 2015 estimated approximately 11,088 practicing otolaryngologists in the United States. Over the next decade, the specialty is on track to suffer from the same shortfall of overall physicians as described by the Association of American Medical Colleges. Current projections have the number of otolaryngologists increasing only by less than 1000 individuals (less than 10% growth) through 2025, assuming current trends in training along with the annual attrition comparable to the overall of 1.7% for all physicians.[8] One of the reasons for such sluggish growth is lack of growth in residency training. Between 2013 and 2017, the number of new residency positions went from 292 to 305, an annual growth rate of only 1.1%.[9] One potential cause for this slow growth, that is not specific to otolaryngology, is that there has been a freeze on Medicare support on graduate medical education since 1997.[10] To cope with this slow growth in the number of otolaryngologists, the field will need to rely on the growth from other midlevel care providers like nurse practitioners, physician assistants, and other support staff. Bureau of Labor Statistics data for nurse practitioners and physician assistants show strong growth at 35% and 30%, respectively, but those numbers are overall and not specific to this field.[7]

GERIATRIC OTOLARYNGOLOGY

As aging occurs, it is commonly associated with increased susceptibility to diseases and in turn an increased demand for medical and surgical services. Many biological mechanisms underlie this impairment in physiology, including oxidative stress, protein and lipid deposits on various cell types, dysregulation or mutations of DNA, increased inflammatory markers, the mortality of somatic stem cells, and decreased response and cell signaling in the immune system, among many others. Ultimately, over time, many organ systems begin to function less efficiently compared with organs of younger ages.[11] This decline becomes clinically evident through routine medical testing, but with older adults, they are also assessed for cognitive abilities along with self-care capacity through activities of daily living (ADLs) and instrumental ADLs.

Frailty is a marker for potential adverse health outcomes, and, depending on various definitions, approximately 15% of older adults in the United States are considered frail.[12] One definition by Fried and colleagues[13] considers a phenotypic frailty as 3 or more of the following: unintentional weight loss (10 lb in past year), self-reported exhaustion, weakness (grip strength), slow walking speed, and low physical activity. Frailty independently predicts falls, worsening mobility or ADLs, hospitalization, and death.[13] Another model, recreated by Rockwood, relies on the accumulative effect of 36 deficits ranging from medical diagnosis to cognitive impairments to emotional states. This theory states that more deficits corresponded with increased frailty and decreased survival probability.[14] More specifically related to surgical outcomes, Makary and colleagues[15] found that frailty independently predicts for postoperative complications, length of stay in the hospital, and discharges to skilled facilities.

Aging is associated with sensory loss across several modalities, and this is an area that will have an enormous impact in otolaryngology given that olfaction, taste, and hearing fall within its purview. Epidemiologic studies in the late 1990s in Beaver Dam, Wisconsin, examined the prevalence of specific sensory losses. Smell impairment (tested with the San Diego Odor Identification Test) rose dramatically with age and had a predominance in men. More than 40% of men in their 70s had smell impairment, whereas only slightly more than 20% of women suffered from this sensory impairment. These numbers jumped to 69% and 59% in men and women, respectively, over the age of 80 years. In the National Health and Nutrition Examination Survey, self-reported taste problems were less than 2% for older adults,[16] although prevalence studies using objective testing in other data sets show that this is also common. In Beaver Dam, more than 3000 participants were assessed for hearing loss, which is defined by an average loss of greater than 25 dB on audiometry testing in a sound booth across frequencies between 500 Hz z and 4000 Hz. They found hearing loss in 43.8%, 66.0%, and 90.0% in the age groups 60 to 69 years, 70 to 79 years, and 80 years or greater, respectively.[17] Higher numbers were found in men across all age ranges. The National Health and Nutritional Examination Surveys from the 2000s yielded slightly lower but similar prevalence of hearing loss of 26.8%, 55.1%, and 79.1% for the same age groups, respectively.[18] Given this high prevalence, Pinto and colleagues[19] used data from the National Social Life, Health, and Aging Project to assess the burden on individuals between the ages of 62 and 90 years. They also found that men reported more hearing loss than women, which is consistent with the results discussed previously. Furthermore, despite that 13% of participants used hearing aids, there was significant burden, with 20% having frustration talking to family members and 42% having trouble with whispered words.

Given these physical and sensory changes in older adults, there are specific disease processes in otolaryngology that will be affected with the demographics shift going forward. The following are a few clinical problems. Presbycusis is highly prevalent, as described previously, and usually affects the higher frequencies of sound. Some of the major physiologic causes of this age-related change include atrophic changes in the basal turn of the cochlea and reduction of neurons.[20] There are, however, additionally many other reasons for hearing loss with aging, including medication side effects, noise exposure, and vascular disease, to name a few. Balance issues also affect older adults. Although ataxia and falls are multifactorial, patients are often under the care of an otolaryngologist to assess vestibular function. Similar to that of the auditory system, the vestibular system also suffers from loss of hair cells, particularly in the ampulla, along with significant neuronal loss.[21] Presbylarynx is evident with a change in vocal quality with aging: men may experience an increased pitch whereas women may experience a lower-pitched and tremulous voice. Several changes can be found within the larynx, such as atrophy of the laryngeal muscles, ossification of the cartilages, decreased collagen and elastin fibers, and edema or polypoid degeneration on the vocal cords.[22] Swallowing disorders can pose a serious health risk for older adults. With aging, there is a decline in sensory discrimination in the oral cavity, pharynx, and supraglottis, which may be a contributing factor to dysphagia and potential aspiration.[23] This can lead to significant morbidity, because respiratory infections are known to be a leading infectious cause for hospitalizations from nursing homes.[24] As the population of older adults increases, estimates of head and neck cancer in this population will rise proportionally. Studies have shown that this type of cancer will increase from 19,000 cases in 2010 for people over 65 years to 31,000 cases in 2030.[25] Another process that will need to be addressed is the aging face, because skin inevitably changes due to years of gravity, ultraviolet sun damage, and contraction of facial musculature, among other factors. There has already been a focus on the safety of cosmetic surgery in older adults, and early studies have shown comparably low complications to that of younger patients.[26]

CONTINUED GROWTH IN DEMAND OF OTOLARYNGOLOGY SERVICES

Given the need for practitioners to care for this growing number of older patients and the large number of conditions for these patients who fall under the specialty, large increases in the demand for otolaryngologists with expertise in caring for older adults are anticipated. Many leaders in the field are cognizant of this reality and have focused on geriatric care as evident by the formation of the American Society of Geriatric Otolaryngology a decade ago,[27] along with new textbooks[11,28,29] and an emerging literature in recent years. When looking at the number of publications found on PubMed regarding geriatric otolaryngology, there has been in an increase from 7 in 2011 to 88 in 2016 (**Fig. 1**). Although the anticipated demographic change in the patient landscape is well known, the specific breakdown of geriatric patients and needed

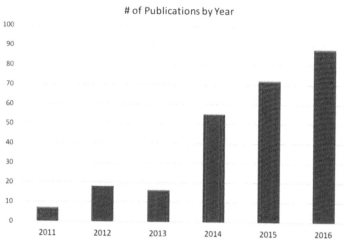

Fig. 1. The number of publications found on PubMed by year with advanced search of geriatric and its synonyms along with otolaryngology and its synonyms.

services in otolaryngology have had little attention in literature. Creighton and colleagues[30] sought to find out the exact characteristics of the population of older adults in a large group practice in Georgia. Between the years 2004 and 2010, they found that the portion of their patients over the age of 65 years jumped from 14.3% to 17.9%. Given the ongoing retirement of the baby boomers, this portion of their practice is estimated to grow to 29.8% by 2030. Another distinguishing characteristic with regard to these visits from patients over 65 years of age is that a vast majority, at 73%, are focused on otology complaints. The top 5 diagnoses in this age group were otology related.

To address this deficit in knowledge, Bhattacharyya and colleagues[31] analyzed Medicare claims made in 2012. Among the 8450 otolaryngologists who submitted claims, there were 13.2 million total services, which yields an average of 1567 services billed per provider in that year. The 3 most popular in office procedures excluding allergy services were the following: removing impacted cerumen performed 700,000 times; diagnostic laryngoscopy performed 550,000 times; and nasal endoscopy performed 400,000 times. Given the Census Bureau's expected 3% annualized growth rate of older adults, the total number of services billed could be approximately 22.7 million, with cerumen removal performed more than 1.2 million times a year by 2030. Removing wax, which may be considered relatively simple, may require a major effort, because the otolaryngology workforce is only growing by approximately 1%. Although Medicare claims do not portray the true clinical and logistical demand of caring for older adults, they at least provide an idea of what these patients will need in the future.

WORKFORCE SOLUTIONS FOR THE DEMOGRAPHICS OF THE FUTURE

Although there is no clear single solution to optimize otolaryngology services for this shift in demographics, several opportunities exist. The most straightforward option is to increase the number of training positions for otolaryngologists, but experts have expressed concern given the lack of government support, as evident in the Medicare freeze in graduate medical training funds since 1997. There has been a push to increase medical school enrollment, as evident in a 3.5% increase seen in 2015.[8] There has been no parallel increase, however, in otolaryngology residency positions. Despite this discrepancy, it must be considered that changes to education and training will require years to realize given the time that is required to train new otolaryngologists.

Changing how specialists treat patients is another method to better serve the population of older adults. Over the past 2 decades, this has been an initiative of the American Geriatrics Society, which created the Geriatrics-for-Specialists Initiative that is "designed to increase awareness of and knowledge in the care of older adults" in specialties, such as otolaryngology.[32] There is an 1-specialty collaboration, including otolaryngology, to create specialty specific geriatric curriculum material, board certification focusing on aging, focus on best practice guidelines, and quality metrics for older adults, along with other goals.[33] The society has also created awards, such as the Jahnigen Scholars (now called the Grants for Early Medical/Surgical Specialists' Transition to Aging Research). Recipients have championed significant research for older adults, and from 2002 to 2014, they had received more than $134 million of funding from federal and private sources; 5% of these scholars were in the field of otolaryngology.[34]

Another solution is to focus on specialty training for advance practice clinicians, like nurse practitioners and physician assistants. According to a study of US data from 2008 and 2009, only 6.3% of ambulatory otolaryngology patients had appointments with advance practice clinicians. There is definitely room to grow this area of practice, because only 0.2% of all nurse practitioners and 0.9% of all physician assistants work in otolaryngology practices. As a comparison, 1.2% of all physicians are otolaryngologists.[35]

This demographic shift yields a unique and exciting opportunity to provide both expedient and cost-efficient care to a growing patient population. Ultimately, whether it is through changes to practices or the workforce or a combination of both, the hope is that it will be sufficient to absorb some of the inevitable strain that the population of older adults will place on the field of otolaryngology in the coming years.

REFERENCES

1. United States Census Bureau. Population Data 2005, 2010, 2012, 2015. Available at: https://www.census.gov/topics/population.html. Accessed September 9, 2017.
2. United Nations: Department of Economic and Social Affairs. Profiles of ageing. Available at: https://esa.un.org/unpd/popdev/Profilesofageing2015/index.html. Accessed September 9, 2017.
3. United States Census Bureau. Projections of the population by sex and selected age groups for the United States: 2015 to 2060. Available at: https://www.census.gov/data/tables/2014/demo/popproj/2014-summary-tables.html. Accessed September 14, 2017.
4. Institute of Medicine. Retooling for an aging America: building the health care workforce. Washington, DC: The National Academies Press; 2008.
5. Congressional Budget Office. The budget and economic outlook: 2017 to 2027. Available at: https://www.cbo.gov/publication/52370. Accessed September 9, 2017.
6. Association of American Medical Colleges. The 2017 update: complexities of physician supply and demand: projections from 2015 to 2030. Available at: https://www.aamc.org/data/workforce/. Accessed September 10, 2017.
7. Bureau of Labor Statistics. Occupational outlook handbook: fastest growing occupations. Available at: https://www.bls.gov/ooh/fastest-growing.htm. Accessed September 9, 2017.

8. Hughes CA, McMenamin P, Mehta V, et al. Otolaryngology workforce analysis. Laryngoscope 2016;126:S5–11.

9. National Resident Matching Program. Results and data: 2017 main residency match. Available at: http://www.nrmp.org/main-residency-match-data/. Accessed September 10, 2017.

10. Association of American Medical Colleges. Graduate medical training: training tomorrow's workforce. Available at: https://www.aamc.org/data/workforce/. Accessed September 10, 2017.

11. Sataloff RT, Johns MM III, Kost KM. Geriatric otolaryngology. New York: Thieme; 2015.

12. Walston JD. Frailty. In: Burton JR, Lee AG, Potter JF, editors. Geriatrics for specialists. Switzerland: Springer International; 2017. p. 3–12.

13. Fried LP, Tangen CM, Walston J, et al. Frailty in older adults: evidence for a phenotype. J Gerontol A Biol Sci Med Sci 2001;56(3):M146–56.

14. Song X, Mitnitski A, Rockwood K. Prevalence and 10-year out- comes of frailty in older adults in relation to deficit accumulation. J Am Geriatr Soc 2010;58(4):681–7.

15. Makary MA, Segev DL, Pronovost PJ, et al. Frailty as a predictor of surgical outcomes in older patients. J Am Coll Surg 2010;210:901–8.

16. Hoffman HJ, Cruickshanks KJ, Davis B. Perspectives on population-based epidemiological studies of olfactory and taste impairment. Ann N Y Acad Sci 2009;1170:514–30.

17. Cruickshanks KJ, Wiley TL, Tweed TS, et al. Prevalence of hearing loss in older adults in Beaver Dam, Wisconsin. The epidemiology of hearing loss study. Am J Epidemiol 1998;148:879–86.

18. Lin FR, Kiparko JK, Ferrucci L. Hearing loss prevalence in the United States. Arch Intern Med 2011;171(20):1851–2.

19. Pinto JM, Kern DW, Wroblewski KE, et al. Sensory function: insights from wave 2 of the national social life, health, and aging project. J Gerontol B Psychol Sci Soc Sci 2014;69(8):S144–53.

20. Schuknecht HF. Presbycusis. Laryngoscope 1955;65:402–19.

21. Konrad HR, Girardi M, Helfert R. Balance and aging. Laryngoscope 1999;109(9):1454–60.

22. Bailey BJ. Geriatric otolaryngology. In: Bailey BJ, Johnson JT, Newlands SD, editors. Head & neck surgery – otolaryngology. Philadelphia: Lippincott Williams & Wilkins; 2006.

23. Aviv JE, Martin JH, Jones ME, et al. Age-related changes in pharyngeal and supraglottic sensation. Ann Otol Rhinol Laryngol 1994;103(10):749–52.

24. Irvine PW, Van Buren N, Crossley K. Causes of hospitalization of nursing home residents: the role of infection. J Am Geriatr Soc 1984;32(2):103–7.

25. Smith BD, Smith GL, Hurria A. Future of cancer incidence in the United States: burdens upon an aging, changing nation. J Clin Oncol 2009;27:2758–65.

26. Veslev M, Gupta V, Winocour J, et al. Safety of cosmetic procedures in the elderly and octogenarian patients. Aesthet Surg J 2015;35(7):864–73.

27. Chalian AA. Accomplishment and opportunity in geriatric otolaryngology. Ear Nose Throat J 2009;88:1156–61.

28. Burton JR, Lee AG, Potter JF. Geriatrics for specialists. Switzerland: Springer International; 2017.

29. Makiyma K, Hirano S. Aging voice. Singapore: Springer International; 2017.

30. Creighton FX Jr, Poliashenko SM, Statham MM, et al. The growing geriatric otolaryngology patient population: a study of 131,700 new patient encounters. Laryngoscope 2013;123:97–102.

31. Bhattacharyya N, Lin HW. Characteristics of otolaryngology claims to medicare in 2012. Otolaryngol Head Neck Surg 2014;151(5):802–4.
32. American Geriatrics Society. Geriatrics for specialists initiative. Available at: http://www.americangeriatrics.org/programs/geriatrics-specialists-initiative. Accessed September 25, 2017.
33. Lee AG, Burton JA, Lundebjerg NE. Geriatrics-for-specialists initiative: an eleven-specialty collaboration to improve care of older adults. J Am Geriatr Soc 2017. https://doi.org/10.1111/jgs.14963.
34. Deiner S. Expanding the field of surgical researchers: the jahnigen career development award. J Am Geriatr Soc 2017. https://doi.org/10.1111/jgs.14967.
35. Bhattacharyya N. Involvement of physician extenders in ambulatory otolaryngology practice. Laryngoscope 2012;122:1010–3.

Age-Related Hearing Loss
Innovations in Hearing Augmentation

Yona Vaisbuch, MD*, Peter Luke Santa Maria, MD, PhD

KEYWORDS

- Presbycusis • Presbyacusis • Age-related hearing loss • Geriatric otology
- Hearing aids • Hearing rehabilitation • Hearing augmentation
- Hearing loss treatment

KEY POINTS

- Age-related hearing loss is a multifactorial condition that effects a major part of the aging population.
- Left untreated, age-related hearing loss can lead to higher risks of cognitive decline, dementia, social isolation, depression, and falls.
- Stigma remains a prominent barriers, so today's devices offer in-the-canal models, miniature size, and camouflage with hair or skin color.
- The mobile era has enabled self-screening, self-fitting, and tele-rehabilitation, and continues to produce other innovations that will potentially improve accessibility.
- Although rigorous scientific efforts have been made in research on inner ear regeneration and some early phase studies exist, the clinical implication remains to be seen.

INTRODUCTION

Age-related hearing loss (ARHL) is the cumulative pathophysiologic changes that occur in hearing attributable to aging. ARHL is also often referred to as "presbycusis" or "presbyacusis."[1] It is typically a progressive, irreversible bilateral symmetric sensorineural high frequency hearing loss (HL).[2] According to the World Health Organization, ARHL is the second most common illness in the geriatric population and is the third most prevalent health condition worldwide.[3] In 2012, based on a review of 42 population-based studies, the World Health Organization estimates were that 328 million adults worldwide had disabling HL (>40 dB in the better hearing ear) and by 2025, with the world population aging, there will be 1.2 billion people over the age of 60, with more than 500 million of them who will suffer significant impairment from

Disclosure: P.L. Santa Maria is a consultant for EarLens. Y. Vaisbuch has nothing to disclose.
Neurotology Division, OHNS Department, Stanford University, 801 Welch Road, Stanford, CA 94305, USA
* Corresponding author.
E-mail address: yona@stanford.edu

ARHL. It affects 1 in 3 persons over the age of 65,[4] and 1 in 2 over the age of 75 in the United States.[5] It is more common in men than women, regardless of occupational or leisure noise exposure.[6,7] Unaddressed HL poses an annual global cost of $750 billion internationally. Direct costs associated include falls and depression; indirect costs include loss of productivity and the quality-adjusted or disability-adjusted life years owing to stigma experienced by individuals with HL, as well as the grief associated with the loss of hearing and the experiences related to the act of hearing or listening.[8] The etiology of ARHL is believed to involve the interaction of multiple factors, including the cochlear degeneration that occurs over time and a genetic predisposition. The primary pathologic findings include hair cells loss, stria vascularis atrophy, and loss of spiral ganglion neurons, as well as changes in the central auditory pathway like atrophy of the gray as well as white matter, changes in the content of some metabolites in the aged brain, and differences between activation of the central auditory system in the young and old brain.[9,10] Other environmental factors can influence the onset and severity of ARHL. These factors include low socioeconomic status, noise exposure, ototoxin exposure (eg, aminoglycosides, chemotherapeutic agents, and heavy metals), infections, smoking, and health comorbidities like hypertension, diabetes, vascular disease, immunologic disorders, and hormonal factors.[11,12] Patients with ARHL often present with difficulty in understanding speech in certain situations, especially in settings with loud background noise such as restaurants or grocery stores. Their families may also report that they start speaking in a louder voice than normal, without the individual being aware of it. Individuals may not present directly for hearing volume complaints, but may primarily seek help for tinnitus or a change in quality of sound, especially an inability to hear high-pitched sounds.[13] The most common interventions in ARHL are hearing augmentation via amplification of sound or direct electrical stimulation of the neural component, via cochlear implantation, when the hearing deterioration is beyond the range of amplification. Both treatments have been shown to be cost effective with the potential to bring great benefit to individuals.[14] There have been recent and emerging innovations in the field of hearing augmentation. In this article, we present an overview of the downstream effects of untreated ARHL. We discuss solutions that are currently available or likely to be available soon based on human clinical trial activity. We also present some new hearing device features that can potentially influence patient experience and satisfaction, which are crucial for adoption and compliance.

LITERATURE REVIEW

Our literature review involved PubMed, Google, and clinicaltrials.gov. The search strategy for PubMed was ("Presbycusis"[MeSH Terms] OR "Presbyacusis"[All-Fields]) OR ("Age Related Hearing Loss"[MeSH Terms] AND "Innovation"[All Fields]) AND ("2007/01/01"[PDAT]: "2017/07/01"[PDAT]). The primary author reviewed all abstracts of studies found with this search strategy. A Google and clinicaltrials.gov search was performed using the following key words: Age related Hearing loss, Presbycusis, Presbyacusis, Geriatric Otology, Hearing augmentation and Innovation. We considered those innovations appropriate for this review as those that are currently available to patients or expected to be available in the near future based on publications and activity in human clinical trials (clinicaltrials.gov).

Age-Related Hearing Loss Sequelae

A large body of evidence is accumulating supporting that ARHL is not only a contributor toward reduced quality of life, but also impacts other physical aspects of aging.

Cognitive decline and dementia

In older adults, cognitive capacity is known to diminish independently with age.[15] Two independent studies using cross-sectional data from the National Health and Nutritional Examination Surveys and the Baltimore Longitudinal Study of Aging, have demonstrated that HL is associated with poorer cognitive functioning on nonverbal tests of memory and executive function among older adults. In both studies, a 25-dB shift in the speech frequency pure tone average was equivalent to nearly 7 years of aging on cognitive scores in older adults. Multiple epidemiology studies have shown that HL is an independent risk factor for the development of dementia.[16–19] One study quantified this by reporting that subjects had 2, 3, and 5 times increased risk for dementia depending on if they had mild, moderate, or severe HL, respectively. Based on this large body of evidence, clinicians should be alert to screening for dementia symptoms within the first 2 years after an ARHL diagnosis.[20] Hearing impaired individuals have been shown to have higher cognitive processing efforts when compared with those with normal hearing, which may increase the severity of other cognitive impairments.[21] Current projections estimate the prevalence of dementia will continue to double every 20 years, such that 1 in every 30 Americans will have dementia by 2050. Attention to HL treatments as prevention is, therefore, critical to addressing the burden of dementia in society.

Work place, social isolation, and depression

HL is often left unrecognized in the early stages. Usually, family members, especially the spouse, are the first to be negatively impacted and bring the problem to attention.[22] Work colleagues also notice the impact of unrecognized HL as it begins to impact work productivity and interpersonal relationships at work. It has been reported that up to 30% of employees have HL, but have not sought care, despite 95% of this group reporting that HL impacts their employment.[23] Unfortunately, little is being done to support seeking care for HL in the workplace environment. A large body of evidence has demonstrated that poor functional hearing is a risk factor for depression in adults.[7,24–29] It is thought that social isolation links HL with depression: the hearing problem causes communication difficulties, which make social interaction challenging, resulting in withdrawal from social engagements and hence a feeling of loneliness and depression. A faster and greater decrease in speech-in-noise recognition is significantly associated with a greater increase in emotional and social isolation.[30,31]

Age-related hearing loss is associated with increased mechanical falls and musculoskeletal injury

The odds of falling are more than doubled in older adults with HL than older adults with normal hearing.[32] A systematic review reported a significant, positive, and independent association between HL and several objective measures of postural control.[33] The severity of HL is directly correlated with increased patient reported difficulty in walking and presentations to the emergency room with long bone fractures.[34] This association may be explained by concomitant dysfunction of both the cochlear and vestibular sense organs given their shared location within the inner ear, decreased auditory cues needed for environmental awareness or cognitive overload, and secondary loss of postural control.[35] HL treatment with hearing aids improve static balance function by reducing the standard deviation velocity. Clinical implications may include improving hearing inputs to increase postural stability in older adults with ARHL.[36]

Innovations in Hearing Augmentation

A summary of the innovations in hearing augmentation is presented in **Table 1**.

Table 1 Innovations in hearing augmentation	
HA sound processing	Feedback cancellation, redirecting frequencies, multidirectional microphones
HA wireless integration	Binaural hearing, CROS, BiCROS, smartphone connectivity, TV streaming, Internet of things, hearables
Reduction in barriers to HA adoption: stigma	Two times smaller size, completely in the canal
Reduction in barriers to HA adoption: comfort	Fitting ear canal mold—3D mold printing, 3D acquisition of mold, soft mold—Eargo
Reduction in barriers to HA adoption—batteries	Rechargeable, 3 mo HA—LYRIC
Reduction in barriers to HA adoption-accessibility	Self-fitting, PSAPs, new legislation toward OTC HA
Photonic driven HA	EarLens
Middle ear partially implantable	Vibrant Soundbridge, Bonebridge, Maxum
Middle ear fully implantable	Carina, Esteem
Bone conduction transcutaneous	BAHA Attract, Sophono, Hearing-glasses, ADHear
CI	MRI compatibility, electroacoustic stimulation, bilateral implants, implants for unilateral deafness, robotic-assisted implantation, steerable electrodes, drug-eluting electrodes
Regenerative and pharmacologic therapies ventures	GENVEC- Ad-Atoh1 gene therapy, DECIBEL THERAPEUTICS, AUDION THERAPEUTICS, Agtc, Auris medical -AM-111

Abbreviations: 3D, 3-dimensional; BiCROS, bilateral microphones with contralateral routing of signal; CI, cochlear implant; CROS, contralateral routing of signal; HA, hearing aid; OTC, over the counter.

New Diagnostic Measures

The method of clinical diagnosis of ARHL has remained the same over 5 decades and involves using pure tone audiometry and word recognition (speech recognition or speech discrimination) in quiet using monosyllabic words. The presence of the noise during the production of speech sounds is disadvantageous for elders, independent of the presence of HL, but having a greater impact for those with HL problems. Several institutes have started to incorporate speech in noise as part of HL workup.[37,38] Efforts are currently being made to either automate the diagnostic process of audiology or put the assessment in the hands of the patient to improve access and to greater identify HL patients in the community. Tools like the Hearing Handicap Inventory for the Elderly Screening version for determining a patient's perception of their HL[39] and self-screening tools that are available online and through mobile apps.[40]

Hearing Aids

Studies have shown that hearing aids provide improved hearing and sustained benefits in hearing and quality of life in the areas of social, emotional, communication, and depression.[41,42] Technological advancement in all areas are being incorporated in hearing aids today.[43] Most patients will benefit from binaural amplification, although it may be a problem in the elderly with auditory processing disorder with binaural interference, making binaural speech perception worse than best hearing ear in monaural mode.[44]

Hearing aids advances in sound processing

Advances have been made on the previous linear mode of amplification across frequencies, including contemporary digital signal processing, which enabled frequency-specific amplification, improved background noise cancellation, improved directionality enabling conversations with multiple speakers, acoustic feedback cancellation, and reduced artifacts. These improvements led to significant improvements in speech perception outcomes in both quiet and noisy environments for adults.[45] One of the next potential advancements is the application of machine learning in speech to individualize and customize signal processing algorithms.[46]

Hearing aids advances in wireless integration

Spatial hearing and performance in noise is improved through better bilateral directionality by incorporating better environmental sensing and multidirectional microphones.[47,48] Wireless technology has also changed the treatment for unilateral HL or single-sided deafness using contralateral routing of signal technology, which transmits sounds from the poorer hearing ear to the better hearing ear by improving the elderly patient usability and satisfaction; and reducing the cumbersome nature of the older wired devices and opening the pathway for bilateral microphones with contralateral routing of signal from the poorer hearing ear to the better hearing ear.[49,50] Wireless technology has also led to the connectivity of hearing aids with other devices. These include connectivity to Smartphones, TV, and music streaming devices and to the "Internet of things" to interact with appliances, door bells and smoke detectors. Better connectivity promotes independence and decreases the need for higher levels of care.[51,52]

Hearing aids reduction in barriers to adoption

The hearing aid global market is dominated by 6 companies (the Big Six), which account for approximately 98% of sales, with an estimated value of $6 billion annually.[53] Despite the huge market, there is still a large untreated population with only an estimated 20% to 25% of those who would benefit from hearing aids.[54] There is also the problem of the delay of presentation with those who finally seek care, coming in at an average age of 71 years.[55] To increase the adoption rate and to decrease the lead time of presentation for care, many strategies are being developed to overcome the barriers for hearing aid adoption, including the associated stigma, perceived complexity of the device, device comfort, and convenience of use, accessibility, and cost.[56–59] To overcome the stigma associated with hearing aids, many design features have been made to make the overall footprint smaller or to hide the receiver in the ear canal. This miniaturization must be balanced with the additional comorbidities in the elderly such as poor vision, reduced manual dexterity, diminished tactile sensitivity, or reduced fine motor coordination.[60,61] The elderly, especially with difficulties in dexterity, find changing hearing aid batteries challenging.[62] Solutions include devices with a rechargeable option. Devices like the Lyric (Phonak-Sonova, Stafa, Switzerland) address this problem and the stigma by placing the entire aid in the canal with no need to replace the device for 3 months.[63] Better comfort and acoustic fit can be achieved through technical improvements that enable better fitting ear mold and vents by using newer imaging of the canal and 3-dimensional mold printing technology.[64,65] Another solution is by designing a noncustom semiopen fitting in the canal device, with a softer ear piece with no need for customized physical fit (EarGo, Mountain View, CA). One current limitation for access is that hearing aids require medical clearance before being dispensed by an official provider. Attempts at removing the need for medical clearance or customization include online purchasing and direct-mail order with simultaneous self-programming. This process enables the end-user to fit and program their own hearing aid.[66] One recent feasibility study of self-programming hearing aids showed that around one-half of patients could successfully insert and fit their hearing aid correctly.[67] In March 2009, the US Food and Drug Administration issued guidance that distinguished devices that amplified sound to treat HL as hearing aids and devices that amplified sound without any intention to treat HL as a personal sound amplifier product (PSAP). This move opened the door for significant market disruption in the industry, making hearing aid technology available without regulation. This brought prices down significantly from the average $3000 per aid to about $20 to $400 per aid, although there is also an accompanying range of quality and safety.[68–72] At the end of 2017, the US government passed a bill creating an over-the-counter hearing aids category.

Assisted Listening Devices

The same advancements in technology that have been implemented in hearing aids have also advanced assisted listening devices.[73–75] An FM system advancements are having significant impact for accessibility in the elderly.[76–79] Another category that has emerged from the consumer electronics industry is Hearables, which combine hearing amplification, hearing protection from noise, and recording of physiologic parameters in the ear transmitted to smartphones[80,81]

Light-Driven Amplification

A novel device for sound amplification was developed by EarLens (Earlens Corporation, Menlo Park, CA), in which amplification is delivered via converting sound into light pulses that drive a customized platform fitted directly onto the umbo. Owing to the elimination of acoustic feedback and a wider range of spectral frequency, the indications for hearing aid fitting can be extended beyond that of traditional hearing aids.[82,83]

Implantable Devices: Active Middle Ear Implants

Active middle ear implants can be divided into the general categories of partially or totally implantable implants using either piezoelectric or electromagnetic systems. Good candidates for active middle ear implants are patients who have structural challenges that prevent traditional hearing aid fitting or who have a large conductive or mixed HL at the limits of traditional hearing aids, but with relatively good preservation of the inner ear.[84] Active middle ear implants are potentially able to drive the ossicular chain directly, resulting in better sound quality. It also increases the amount of gain delivered without feedback. Outcomes with Active middle ear implants in the elderly population as a subgroup have not been reported specifically, but have been documented within the larger adult patient group.[85] In a partially implantable active middle ear implants, the microphone is in a device resembling a conventional hearing aid. The amplified signal is transmitted to drive the middle ear conductive mechanism directly. The Vibrant Soundbridge (Med-El, Innsbruck, Austria) achieves this via transmitting sound to a floating mass transducer, which is a magnet surrounded by an electromagnetic coil, placed onto the ossicular chain or against the round window.[86–88] Whereas the Vibrant Soundbridge has an external component resembling the footprint of a traditional cochlear implant, the Maxum (Ototronix, Houston, TX) microphone and processor is hidden in the canal. The processor stimulates a magnet attached to the stapes superstructure joint. The Maxum can also be inserted under local anesthesia in the office.[89,90] Fully implantable active middle ear implants offer additional lifestyle advantages to partially implantable active middle ear implants such as continuous use at all hours and the ability to get the ear wet.[91,92] Carina (Cochlear, Melbourne, Australia) involves an electromagnetic transducer tip typically attached to a small hole drilled into the incus. All the components are implanted in a manner like a cochlear implant with demonstration of improved functional outcomes.[93,94] The Esteem (Envoy Medical, White Bear Lake, MN) uses piezoelectric transducers made of a crystal aggregate material that has the property of reverse mechanical transduction, to convert movement of the tympanic membrane to overdrive the stapes. The battery that is implanted in the sound processor lasts more than 5 years on average.[95,96] In a study using the patient's contralateral ear as a control, there was significant difference between Esteem and hearing aids in either performance or satisfaction.[97]

Bone-Conducting Hearing Devices

Individuals with ARHL who would benefit from sound amplification but are not able to wear conventional hearing aids, bone conduction hearing aids can be considered. Typical indications include an ipsilateral ear with large conductive HL that cannot be reconstructed or single-sided deafness with normal contralateral hearing ear.[98,99] Usage of percutaneous bone conduction hearing devices (Baha Connect [Cochlear] and the Ponto [Oticon, Copenhagen, Denmark]) started decades ago with patients with bilateral conductive or mixed HL,[100] before being expanded into single-sided deafness,[101] where the outcomes are now excellent. The vast majority (85%) of patients with single-sided deafness continue to use their device 5 years after implantation.[102] Most of the innovation in these devices has been around adopting less invasive techniques and better surgical access (linear and punch incisions) to avoid soft tissue complications that include periabutment dermatitis, poor esthetics, and loss of skin sensation.[103–106] The next innovation in this area was to remove the need for the transcutaneous abutment altogether. Transcutaneous magnetic bone conduction hearing devices (Baha Attract [Cochlear] and SOPHONO [Medtronic, Boulder, CO]) were developed using an internal vibrating component fixed to the skull with a sound processor connected externally via a magnet across the intact skin.[107] A soft pad is used between the skin and the external magnet to distribute pressure over the contact area and decrease skin irritation.[108] The Bonebridge (Med-El) is another partially implanted bone conduction device, except for an external sound processor. There may be an audiological advantage by physically separating the vibrating component from the sound processor through reduced feedback.[109] Benefits also include higher functional gain, better speech perception, and lower rates of cutaneous complications.[110] To avoid surgery altogether an in-the-mouth hearing system, the SoundBite (Sonitus Medical, San Mateo, CA), was developed. The device consisted of an in-the-mouth vibrating device custom fit around the upper molars and a behind-the-ear microphone. Benefits included increased output (up to 30 dB higher), gain (up to 26 dB higher) and patient satisfaction compared with the other bone conduction devices.[111] At the beginning of 2015, the company ceased operations because coverage of this device was restricted.[112] There are also several other bone conductive hearing aids for which surgical intervention is not needed, including hearing glasses or headbands that create firm contact against the skull.[113] The ADHEAR (Med-El) currently under clinical trial is a bone conduction device applied by a single-use adhesive to the skin behind the pinna that can be worn for up to a week and is water resistant. Because noninvasive approaches do not have as firm interface with the cranium, there is a loss of gain when compared with traditional bone anchored hearing aids.[114]

Implantable Devices: Cochlear Implants

As of December 2012, approximately 324,200 registered devices have been implanted worldwide. In the United States, roughly 58,000 devices have been implanted in adults as reported by the 3 main cochlear implant manufacturers (AB [Advance Bionic], Med El, and Cochlear).[115] A new cochlear implant device from Oticon, the Neuro Zti, was recently introduced and is under safety and efficacy clinical trial since the beginning of 2016.[116] Cochlear implants have long been established as effective in elderly populations with comparable speech and quality of life outcomes as in younger patients.[117-121] In addition, complication rates have been shown to be no higher than younger patients if comorbidities are accounted for, except for a small increase in cardiovascular complications and a higher admission rate,[122-124] imbalance, and increased risk of falling after cochlear implantation may be common, particularly in the short term in the elderly.[125,126] Expanding indications for cochlear implants include bilateral implantation for adults,[127,128] less severe loss of hearing before implantation, and single-sided deafness, especially those with significant tinnitus.[129] Cochlear implants for single-sided deafness remains the only option for returning some true binaural hearing with sound localization.[130-132] Because elderly patients often undergo MRI for diagnoses of other diseases, the MRI incompatibility of cochlear implants had previously limited its uptake in some patients or necessitated magnet removal procedure. Now all cochlear implants manufacturers have received US Food and Drug Administration approval for 1.5 T MRI.[133] In addition, the SYNCHRONY Cochlear Implant (Med-El) is designed with a rotatable diametrically magnetized internal self-aligning magnet, allowing for the use of a 3.0 T MRI.[134] Future areas of cochlear implants innovation in development include incorporating a robotic insertion device to minimize insertion trauma.[135] In a clinical study using a robotic system, 8 of 9 patients were successfully implanted using the proposed approach with 6 insertions completely within the scala tympani. Complications in this study included the use of the backup implant after the first electrode was dislodged, tip fold-over, and facial nerve paresis (House-Brackmann II/VI at 12 months) secondary to heat generation during drilling, all show that more development is needed.[136] Drug eluting cochlear implants, incorporating antiinflammatories to preserve residual hearing or neurotrophins to promote growth from the spiral ganglion toward the electrode array stimulus improve neuron–electrode proximity, which could result in lowered electrical stimulation thresholds. Reduced thresholds support the creation of smaller electrode structures and high-density electrode prostheses, greatly enhancing prosthesis control and function, are other areas of research trials.[137-139]

Cochlear implants: electroacoustic stimulation

Electric acoustic stimulation refers to a device that incorporates a hearing aid for the low frequencies and a cochlear implant for the high frequencies.[140] This combined method addresses the specific needs of patients presenting with good low frequency hearing (with normal to moderate sensorineural HL in the low frequencies up to 1500 Hz) but poorer hearing in the high frequencies (sloping to severe-to-profound HL in the high frequencies 2000 Hz and above, preoperative scores for speech understanding for single words in quiet is 60% or less). Despite residual low frequencies, these patients struggle to understand speech. Preservation of the low frequencies leads to greater patient satisfaction, particularly with enjoyment and recognition of music.[141] There is an inherent risk of losing the residual low frequencies with implantation, but those who do, may still benefit from the cochlear implant electrical only condition and overall will report better word recognition and quality of life.[142]

A large field of research has developed around prevention of loss of residual hearing through hearing preservation surgical techniques, pharmaceuticals, and atraumatic electrode design.[143]

Cochlear implants: related technological advances

The sound processing advances in hearing aids are also reflected in the cochlear implants with improved microphone directionality, noise reduction and connectivity to a contra-lateral hearing aid, smartphone and other devices.[144] A potential barrier to cochlear implant adoption can be the mapping process that occurs as part of the post operative rehabilitation. This process can involve many labor-intensive visits with implant audiologists over a year or more. Remote and automated mapping are advances in development looking to improve this factor.[145,146]

Pharmaceutical Preventive Therapies

The research to date suggests that oxidative stress and mitochondrial DNA deletion play a major role in the pathophysiology of ARHL.[147] Several therapies and preventive measures have been studied. At the time of publication of this article, there are no proven preventative measures. It seems that therapeutics strategies targeting only radical oxygen species overproduction is helpful (particularly in laboratory animals) but, is not sufficient to avoid or reduce the effects of aging on hearing.[148] As a result, other strategies have emerged, which mainly include calcium channel blockers,[149] statins,[150] heat shock protein inducer,[151] cochlear vasodilators,[152] salicylate therapy,[153] electrical stimulation to restore the endocochlear potential by enhancement of outer hair cells electromotility,[154] antiapoptotic treatments, and caloric restriction.[155,156] The protective effect of each of these against ARHL has been inconsistent across reports. Auris Medical (Zug, Switzerland) developed intratympanic single treatment of JNK inhibitors to prevent apoptosis through blocking signal transduction for subjects suffering from severe to profound idiopathic sudden sensorineural HL, which is in phase III efficacy and safety trials.[157,158]

Regenerative Therapies: Future Directions

The holy grail of ARHL is restoring function rather than amplifying sound. For the past 30 years, research has provided a better understanding of the mechanisms underlying inner ear development.[159,160] There are several discoveries including avian cochlear hair cell regeneration, pluripotent stem cell differentiation,[161] cell transplantation, the presence of endogenous stem cells, and the potential therapeutic application of gene transfer for HL.[162] Although much has been learned, these approaches are still in the experimental stages. There are many challenges involved in the process of cochlear nerve and hair cell regeneration. Although, to date, there are no clinical trials in this field, several recent discoveries using cell culture and animal models were incorporated in commercial ventures, which give hope that otolaryngologists will have novel, regenerative therapeutic options for the management of ARHL in the future.[163] GENVEC (Gaithersburg, MD) has one phase I human clinical trial using Ad-Atoh1 gene therapy that began at the end of 2014. This gene induces the differentiation of inner ear sensory cells during embryonic development.[164] The drug is delivered through a recombinant adenovirus vector CGF166, which is injected intralabyrinthine. Another approach is taken by DECIBEL THERAPEUTICS (Boston, MA), which is targeting synapse restoration as the main reason for hidden HL and may precede a progressive decline in hearing. AUDION THERAPEUTICS (Amsterdam, the Netherlands) drug development program currently focuses on inner hair cell regeneration through notch inhibition, using new small molecule compounds, which is planned to enter a clinical safety study in patients with HL in 2017. Last, Agtc (Alachua, FL) is expanding its adeno-associated virus technology platform beyond retinal degenerative diseases, to address targets that could help to treat patients with inherited hearing disorders.

Inner Ear Treatments Delivery

The anatomic and pharmacologic inaccessibility of the inner ear is a major challenge in drug-based treatment of ARHL. This factor also makes the pharmacokinetic characterization of new drugs with systemic delivery challenging. Direct delivery of drugs to cochlear fluids bypasses pharmacokinetic barriers and helps to minimize systemic toxicity, but anatomic barriers make administration of multiple doses difficult without an automated delivery system. Such a system may be required for hair cell regeneration treatments, which will likely require timed delivery of several drugs. To address these challenges, a micropump is being developed in animal models for controlled, automated inner ear drug delivery with the goal of producing a long-term implantable/wearable delivery system.[165]

SUMMARY

ARHL is a multifactorial condition that affects a major part of the aging population and, if left untreated, can lead to major health risks. In this article, we covered the temporary and near future conceptual and technological developments in ARHL treatments.

Presently, patients can benefit from improved digital sound processing, photon-driven actuator that is placed on the ear drum, and nonimplantable bone conduction hearing aid. The indications for cochlear implants have broadened as well, making it possible to implant patients with residual low frequency hearing using hybrid cochlear implants technology, unilateral deafness, or implanting both ears in adults. Although rigorous scientific efforts are made in inner ear regeneration and some early phase clinical studies are underway, the clinical implication is still far away. To address untreated ARHL in this era, several measures still need to take place: public campaigns aiming to raise awareness to the downstream effects of untreated ARHL; creating accessible screening and consulting programs for municipalities, institutions, and work places; and targeting caregivers and family members as the facilitators on getting their loved ones to consider hearing augmentation. The mobile era of self-screening, self-fitting, tele-rehabilitation and the upcoming opening of the US market to over-the-counter hearing aids can potentially disrupt the market, with reduced prices worldwide owing to increased competition, which can substantially improve accessibility and affordability.[166] With these innovations mentioned, by reaching more patients and at a younger age, hopefully we will be able to prevent or diminish the downstream effects of untreated ARHL.

REFERENCES

1. National Center for Biotechnology Information. Presbycusis (age-related hearing loss). Available at: https://www.ncbi.nlm.nih.gov/pubmedhealth/PMHT0024983/. Accessed October 5, 2017.
2. Huang Q, Tang J. Age-related hearing loss or presbycusis. Eur Arch Otorhinolaryngol 2010;267(8):1179–91.
3. Cruickshanks KJ, Wiley TL, Tweed TS, et al. Prevalence of hearing loss in older adults in Beaver Dam, Wisconsin. The Epidemiology of Hearing Loss Study. Am J Epidemiol 1998;148(9):879–86.

4. Roth TN, Hanebuth D, Probst R. Prevalence of age-related hearing loss in Europe: a review. Eur Arch Otorhinolaryngol 2011;268(8):1101–7.
5. Lin FR, Niparko JK, Ferrucci L. Hearing loss prevalence in the United States. Available at: https://www.ncbi.nlm.nih.gov/pmc/articles/PMC3564588/. Accessed March 12, 2017.
6. Yamasoba T, Lin FR, Someya S, et al. Current concepts in age-related hearing loss: epidemiology and mechanistic pathways. Hear Res 2013;303:30–8.
7. Agrawal Y, Platz EA, Niparko JK. Prevalence of hearing loss and differences by demographic characteristics among US adults: data from the National Health and Nutrition Examination Survey, 1999-2004. Arch Intern Med 2008;168(14): 1522–30.
8. Global costs of unaddressed hearing loss and cost-effectiveness of interventions: a WHO report, 2017. Geneva: World Health Organization; 2017.
9. Schuknecht HF, Gacek MR. Cochlear pathology in presbycusis. Ann Otol Rhinol Laryngol 1993;102:1–16.
10. Ouda L, Profant O, Syka J. Age-related changes in the central auditory system. Cell Tissue Res 2015;361(1):337–58.
11. Momi SK, Wolber LE, Fabiane SM, et al. Genetic and environmental factors in age-related hearing impairment. Twin Res Hum Genet 2015;18(4):383–92.
12. Tan HE, Lan NSR, Knuiman MW, et al. Associations between cardiovascular disease and its risk factors with hearing loss-A cross-sectional analysis. Clin Otolaryngol 2018;43(1):172–81.
13. World Health Organization (WHO). Age-related hearing loss (presbycusis). Available at: http://www.who.int/features/qa/83/en/. Accessed October 12, 2017.
14. Contrera KJ, Wallhagen MI, Mamo SK, et al. Hearing loss health care for older adults. J Am Board Fam Med 2016;29(3):394–403.
15. Lin FR, Yaffe K, Xia J, et al, Health ABC Study Group. Hearing loss and cognitive decline in older adults. JAMA Intern Med 2013;173(4):293–9.
16. Lin FR, Metter EJ, O'Brien RJ, et al. Hearing loss and incident dementia. Arch Neurol 2011;68(2):214–20.
17. Lin FR. Hearing loss and cognition among older adults in the United States. J Gerontol A Biol Sci Med Sci 2011;66(10):1131–6.
18. Thomson RS, Auduong P, Miller AT, et al. Hearing loss as a risk factor for dementia: a systematic review. Laryngoscope Investig Otolaryngol 2017;2:69–79.
19. Golub JS, Luchsinger JA, Manly JJ, et al. Observed hearing loss and incident dementia in multiethnic cohort. J Am Geriatr 2017;65:1691–7.
20. Su P, Hsu CC, Lin HC, et al. Age related hearing loss and dementia: a 10 year national population based study. Eur Arch Otolaryngol 2017;274:2327–34.
21. Golub JS. Brain changes associated with age-related hearing loss. Curr Opin Otolaryngol Head Neck Surg 2017;25(5):347–52.
22. Dawes P, Emsley R, Cruickshanks KJ, et al. Hearing loss and cognition: the role of hearing aids, social isolation and depression. PLoS One 2015;10(3): e0119616.
23. Productivity threat: 25%+ U.S. workers have untreated hearing loss. Available at: https://www.epichearing.com/blog/silent-threat-productivity-untreated-hearing-loss-impacts-one-four-u-s-workers/. Accessed October 12, 2017.
24. Hsu WT, Hsu CC, Wen MH, et al. Increased risk of depression in patients with acquired sensory hearing loss: a 12-year follow-up study. Medicine (Baltimore) 2016;95(44):e5312.

25. Carabellese C, Appollonio I, Rozzini R, et al. Sensory impairment and quality of life in a community elderly population. J Am Geriatr Soc 1993;41(4):401–7.

26. Kramer SE, Kapteyn TS, Kuik DJ, et al. The association of hearing impairment and chronic diseases with psychosocial health status in older age. J Aging Health 2002;14(1):122–37.

27. Dalton DS, Cruickshanks KJ, Klein BE, et al. The impact of hearing loss on quality of life in older adults. Gerontologist 2003;43(5):661–8.

28. Gopinath B, Hickson L, Schneider J, et al. Hearing-impaired adults are at increased risk of experiencing emotional distress and social engagement restrictions five years later. Age Ageing 2012;41(5):618–23.

29. Saito H, Nishiwaki Y, Michikawa T, et al. Hearing handicap predicts the development of depressive symptoms after 3 years in older community-dwelling Japanese. J Am Geriatr Soc 2010;58(1):93–7.

30. Pronk M, Deeg DJ, Smits C, et al. Hearing loss in older persons: does the rate of decline affect psychosocial health? J Aging Health 2014;26(5):703–23.

31. Mick P, Kawachi I, Lin FR. The association between hearing loss and social isolation in older adults. Otolaryngol Head Neck Surg 2014;150(3):378–84.

32. Jiam NT, Li C, Agrawal Y. Hearing loss and falls: a systematic review and meta-analysis. Laryngoscope 2016;126(11):2587–96.

33. Agmon M, Lavie L, Doumas M. The association between hearing loss, postural control, and mobility in older adults: a systematic review. J Am Acad Audiol 2017;28(6):575–88.

34. Woollacott M, Shumway-Cook A. Attention and the control of posture and gait: a review of an emerging area of research. Gait Posture 2002;16(1):1–14.

35. Lin FR, Ferrucci L, Metter EJ, et al. Hearing loss and cognition in the Baltimore Longitudinal Study of Aging. Neuropsychology 2011;25(6):763–70.

36. Negahban H, Bavarsad Cheshmeh Ali M, Nassadj G. Effect of hearing aids on static balance function in elderly with hearing loss. Gait Posture 2017;58:126–9.

37. Vermiglio AJ, Soli SD, Freed DJ, et al. The relationship between high-frequency pure-tone hearing loss, hearing in noise test (HINT) thresholds, and the articulation index. J Am Acad Audiol 2012;23(10):779–88.

38. Boboshko MY, Golovanova LE, Zhilinskaia EV, et al. Speech intelligibility in elderly hearing impaired people. Adv Gerontol 2016;29(4):663–9.

39. Weinstein B. Geriatric audiology. 2nd edition. New York: Thieme; 2013.

40. Abu-Ghanem S, Handzel O, Ness L, et al. Smartphone-based audiometric test for screening hearing loss in the elderly. Eur Arch Otorhinolaryngol 2016;273(2): 333–9.

41. Giroud N, Lemke U, Reich P, et al. The impact of hearing aids and age related hearing loss on auditory plasticity across three month – an electrical neuroimaging study. Hearing Res 2017;353:162–75.

42. Mulrow CD, Tuley MR, Aguilar C. Sustained benefits of hearing aids. J Speech Hear Res 1992;35(6):1402–5.

43. Ferguson MA, Kitterick PT, Chong LY, et al. Hearing aids for mild to moderate hearing loss in adults. Cochrane Database Syst Rev 2017;(9):CD012023.

44. Jerger J, Silman S, Lew HL, et al. Case studies in binaural interference: covering evidence from behavioral and electrophysiologic measures. J Am Acad Audiol 1993;4(2):122–31.

45. Ellis RJ, Munro KJ. Benefit from, and acclimatization to, frequency compression hearing aids in experienced adult hearing-aid users. Int J Audiol 2015;54(1): 37–47.

46. Zhang T, Mustiere F, Micheyl C. Intelligent hearing aids: the next revolution. Conf Proc IEEE Eng Med Biol Soc 2016;2016:72–6.

47. Ibrahim I, Parsa V, Macpherson E, et al. Evaluation of speech intelligibility and sound localization abilities with hearing aids using binaural wireless technology. Audiol Res 2012;3(1):e1.

48. Neher T, Wagener KC, Latzel M. Speech reception with different bilateral directional processing schemes: influence of binaural hearing, audiometric asymmetry, and acoustic scenario. Hear Res 2017;353:36–48.

49. Williams VA, McArdle RA, Chisolm TH. Subjective and objective outcomes from new BiCROS technology in a veteran sample. J Am Acad Audiol 2012;23(10): 789–806.

50. Oeding K, Valente M. Sentence recognition in noise and perceived benefit of noise reduction on the receiver and transmitter sides of a BICROS hearing aid. J Am Acad Audiol 2013;10:980–91.

51. Unwin BK, Andrews CM, Andrews PM, et al. Therapeutic home adaptations for older adults with disabilities. Am Fam Physician 2009;80(9):963–8.

52. Domingo MC. An overview of the Internet of Things for people with disabilities. J Netw Comput Appl 2012;35(2):584–96.

53. Blustein J, Weinstein BE. Opening the market for lower cost hearing aids: regulatory change can improve the health of older Americans. Am J Public Health 2016;106(6):1032–5.

54. Kochkin S. MarkeTrak VIII: 25 years trends in the hearing health market. Hearing Rev 2009;16(11):12–31.

55. Bisgaard N, Ruf S. Findings from Eurotrak surveys from 2009 to 2015: hearing loss prevalence, hearing aid adoption, and benefits of hearing aid use. Am J Audiol 2017;26(3S):451–61.

56. Wallhagen MI. The stigma of hearing loss. Gerontologist 2010;50(1):66–75.

57. Barker AB, Leighton P, Ferguson MA. Coping together with hearing loss: a qualitative meta-synthesis of the psychosocial experiences of people with hearing loss and their communication partners. Int J Audiol 2017;56(5):297–305.

58. Kochkin S. MarkeTrak VII: obstacles to adult non-user adoption of hearing aids. Hearing Jour 2007;60(4):27–43.

59. Kochkin S. MarkeTrak VIII: the key influencing factors in hearing aid purchase intent. Hear Rev 2012;19(3):12–25.

60. Tonning F, Warland A, Tonning K. Hearing instruments for the elderly hearing impaired. A comparison of in-the-canal and behind-the-ear hearing instruments in first-time users. Scand Audiol 1991;20(1):69–74.

61. Humes LE, Wilson DL, Humes AC. Examination of differences between successful and unsuccessful elderly hearing aid candidates matched for age, hearing loss and gender. Int J Audiol 2003;42(7):432–41.

62. Singh G, Pichora-Fuller MK, Hayes D, et al. The aging hand and the ergonomics of hearing aid controls. Ear Hear 2013;34(1):e1–13.

63. PHONAK. Lyric 3 product information. Available at: https://www.phonakpro. com/content/dam/phonakpro/gc_hq/en/products_solutions/hearing_aid/lyric/ documents/product_information_lyric3_027-0152.pdf. Accessed October 12, 2017.

64. Stevenson D, Searchfield G, Xu X. Spatial design of hearing AIDS incorporating multiple vents. Trends Hear 2014;21:18.

65. Lantos Technologies. 3D ear scanning. Available at: http://www.lantostechnologies. com/. Accessed October 12, 2017.

66. Manchaiah V, Taylor B, Dockens AL, et al. Application of direct to consumer hearing devices for adults with hearing loss: a review. Clin Interv Aging 2017; 12:859–71.

67. Convery E, Keidser G, Seeto M, et al. Evaluation of the self-fitting process with a commercially hearing aid. J Am Acad Audiol 2017;28(2):109–18.

68. Smith C, Wilber LA, Cavitt K. PSAps vs hearing aids: an electroacoustic analysis of performance and fitting capabilities. Hear Rev 2016;23(7):18.

69. Stamp E. The pros and cons of PSAPs. Hearing Health (Spring); 2016. p. 20–2.

70. Mamo SK, Reed NS, Nieman CL, et al. Personal sound amplifiers for adults with hearing loss. Am J Med 2016;129(3):245–50.

71. McPherson B, Wong ET. Effectiveness of an affordable hearing aid with elderly persons. Disabil Rehabil 2005;27(11):601–9.

72. Sacco G, Gonfrier S, Teboul B, et al. Clinical evaluation of an over the counter hearing aid (TEO First) in elderly patients suffering of mild to moderate hearing loss. BMC Geriatr 2016;9(16):136.

73. Wittich W, Southall K, Johnson A. Usability of assistive listening devices by older adults with low vision. Disabil Rehabil Assist Technol 2016;11(7):564–71.

74. Kim JS, Kim CH. A review of assistive listening device and digital wireless technology for hearing instruments. Korean J Audiol 2014;18(3):105–11.

75. Lopez EA, Costa OA, Ferrari DV. Development and technical validation of the mobile based assistive listening system: a smartphone-based remote microphone. Am J Audiol 2016;25(3S):288–94.

76. Kam AC, Sung JK, Lee T, et al. Improving mobile phone speech recognition by personalized amplification: application in people with normal hearing and mild to moderate hearing loss. Ear Hear 2017;38(2):e85–92.

77. Crandall C, Smaldino J. Room acoustics and amplification. In: Valente M, Roeser R, Hosford-Dunn H, editors. Audiology: treatment strategies. New York: Thieme Medical Publishers; 2000. p. 601–37.

78. Chisolm TH, Noe CM, McArdle R, et al. Evidence for the use of hearing assistive technology by adults: the role of the FM system. Trends Amplif 2007;11:73–89.

79. Stika C, Ross M, Ceuvas C. Hearing aid services and satisfaction: the consumer viewpoint. Hear Loss 2002;23:25–31.

80. Taylor B. Hearables: the morphing of hearing aids consumer electronic devices. Audiol Today 2015;27(6):22–30.

81. Hunn N. The market for hearable devices 2016-2020: a consumer centric approach. London: WiForce Wireless consulting; 2016. Available at: http://www.nickhunn.com. Accessed August 30, 2017.

82. Gantz BJ, Perkins R, Murray M, et al. Light-driven contact hearing aid for broad-spectrum amplification: safety and effectiveness pivotal study. Otol Neurotol 2017;38(3):352–9.

83. Puria S, Maria PL, Perkins R. Temporal-bone measurements of the maximum equivalent pressure output and maximum stable gain of a light-driven hearing system that mechanically stimulates the umbo. Otol Neurotol 2016;37(2):160–6.

84. Wagner F, Todt I, Wagner J, et al. Indications and candidacy for active middle ear implants. Adv Otorhinolaryngol 2010;69:20–6.

85. Carlson ML, Pelosi S, Haynes DS. Historical development of active middle ear implants. Otolaryngol Clin North Am 2014;47(6):893–914.

86. Arthur D. The vibrant® soundbridge™. Trends Amplif 2002;6(2):67–72.

87. Lüers JC, Hüttenbrink KB. Vibrant Soundbridge rehabilitation of conductive and mixed hearing loss. Otolaryngol Clin North Am 2014;47(6):915–26.

88. Luetje CM, Brackman D, Balkany TJ, et al. Phase III clinical trial results with the Vibrant Soundbridge implantable middle ear hearing device: a prospective controlled multicenter study. Otolaryngol Head Neck Surg 2002;126:97–107.
89. Pelosi S, Carlson ML, Glasscock ME. Implantable hearing devices: the ototronix MAXUM system. Otolaryngol Clin North Am 2014;47(6):953–65.
90. Hunter JB, Carlson ML, Glasscock ME. The ototronix MAXUM middle ear implant for severe high-frequency sensorineural hearing loss: preliminary results. Laryngoscope 2016;126(9):2124–7.
91. Jenkins HA, Uhler K. Otologics active middle ear implants. Otolaryngol Clin North Am 2014;47(6):967–78.
92. Lim HG, Kim JH, Shin DH, et al. Wireless charging pillow for a fully implantable hearing aid: design of a circular array coil based on finite element analysis for reducing magnetic weak zones. Biomed Mater Eng 2015;26:S1741–7.
93. Bruschini L, Forli F, Santoro A, et al. Fully implantable Otologics MET Carina device for the treatment of sensorineural hearing loss. Preliminary surgical and clinical results. Acta Otorhinolaryngol Ital 2009;29(2):79–85.
94. Bruschini L, Berrettini S, Forli F, et al. The Carina© middle ear implant: surgical and functional outcomes. Eur Arch Otorhinolaryngol 2016;273(11):3631–40.
95. Maurer J, Savvas E. The Esteem System: a totally implantable hearing device. Adv Otorhinolaryngol 2010;69:59–71.
96. Marzo SJ, Sappington JM, Shohet JA. The Envoy Esteem implantable hearing system. Otolaryngol Clin North Am 2014;47(6):941–52.
97. Monini S, Biagini M, Atturo F, et al. Esteem® middle ear device versus conventional hearing aids for rehabilitation of bilateral sensorineural hearing loss. Eur Arch Otorhinolaryngol 2013;270(7):2027–33.
98. Mudry A, Tjellström A. Historical background of bone conduction hearing devices and bone conduction hearing aids. Adv Otorhinolaryngol 2011;71:1–9.
99. Van Barneveld DCPBM, Kok HJW, Noten JFP, et al. Determining fitting ranges of various bone conduction hearing aids. Clin Otolaryngol 2018;43(1):68–75.
100. Syms MJ, Hernandez KE. Bone conduction hearing: device auditory capability to aid in device selection. Otolaryngol Head Neck Surg 2014;150(5):866–71.
101. Yuen HW, Bodmer D, Smilsky K, et al. Management of single-sided deafness with the bone-anchored hearing aid. Otolaryngol Head Neck Surg 2009;141:16–23.
102. Kompis M, Wimmer W, Caversaccio M. Long term benefit of bone anchored hearing systems in single sided deafness. Acta Otolaryngol 2017;137(4):398–402.
103. Brant JA, Gudis D, Ruckenstein MJ. Results of Baha® implantation using a small horizontal incision. Am J Otolaryngol 2013;34(6):641–5.
104. Calon TG, van Hoof M, van den Berge H, et al. Minimally Invasive Ponto Surgery compared to the linear incision technique without soft tissue reduction for bone conduction hearing implants: study protocol for a randomized controlled trial. Trials 2016;17(1):540.
105. Dun CA, Faber HT, de Wolf MJ, et al. An overview of different systems: the bone-anchored hearing aid. Adv Otorhinolaryngol 2011;71:22–31.
106. Sardiwalla Y, Jufas N, Morris DP. Direct cost comparison of minimally invasive punch technique versus traditional approaches for percutaneous bone anchored hearing devices. J Otolaryngol Head Neck Surg 2017;46(1):46.
107. Dimitriadis PA, Hind D, Wright K, et al. Single-center experience of over a hundred implantations of a transcutaneous bone conduction device. Otol Neurotol 2017;38(9):1301–7.

108. Cooper T, McDonald B, Ho A. Passive Transcutaneous bone conduction hearing implants: a systematic review. Otol Neurotol 2017;38(9):1225–32.

109. Riss D, Arnoldner C, Baumgartner WD, et al. Indication criteria and outcomes with the Bonebridge transcutaneous bone-conduction implant. Laryngoscope 2014;124(12):2802–6.

110. Bento RF, Lopes PT, Cabral Junior Fda C. Bonebridge bone conduction implant. Int Arch Otorhinolaryngol 2015;19(4):277–8.

111. Gurgel RK, Shelton C. The SoundBite hearing system: patient-assessed safety and benefit study. Laryngoscope 2013;123(11):2807–12.

112. The Hearing Review. Sonitus Medical to hold auction after closing its doors. Available at: http://www.hearingreview.com/2015/02/sonitus-medical-holds-auction-closing-doors. Accessed October 12, 2017.

113. Greenberg JE, Desloge JG, Zurek PM. Evaluation of array-processing algorithms for a headband hearing aid. J Acoust Soc Am 2003;113(3):1646–57.

114. Use of ADHEAR, a non-implantable bone conduction hearing system, in children with single sided deafness and/or conductive hearing loss. Available at: https://clinicaltrials.gov/ct2/show/NCT03327194. Accessed October 12, 2017.

115. National Institute on Deafness and Other Communication Disorder. What does the future hold for cochlear implants? Available at:https://www.nidcd.nih.gov/health/cochlear-implants#e. Accessed October 12, 2017.

116. Available at:https://clinicaltrials.gov/NCT02941627. Accessed October 12, 2017.

117. Ching TYC, Dillon H, Byrne D. Speech recognition of hearing-impaired listeners: predictions from audibility and the limited role of high-frequency amplification. J Acoust Soc Am 1998;103:1128–40.

118. Coelho DH, McKinnon BJ. Regenerative Cochlear implantation in elderly. In: Sataloff RT, Johns MM, Kost KM, editors. Geriatric Otolaryngology. 2015. p. 63–76.

119. Waltzman SB, Cohen NL, Shapiro WH. The benefits of cochlear implantation in the geriatric population. Otolaryngol Head Neck Surg 1993;108:329–33.

120. Sonnet MH, Montaut-Verient B, Niemier JY, et al. Cognitive abilities and quality of life after cochlear implantation in the elderly. Otol Neurotol 2017;38(8):e296–301.

121. Francis HW, Chee N, Yeagle J, et al. Impact of cochlear implants on the functional health status of older adults. Laryngoscope 2002;112:1482–8.

122. Coelho DH, Yeh J, Kim JT, et al. Cochlear implantation is associated with minimal anesthetic risk in the elderly. Laryngoscope 2009;119(2):355–8.

123. Kelsall DC, Shallop JK, Burnelli T. Cochlear implantation in the elderly. Am J Otol 1995;16:609–15.

124. Carlson ML, Breen JT, Gifford RH, et al. Cochlear implantation in the octogenarian and nonagenarian. Otol Neurotol 2010;31(8):1343–9.

125. Stevens MN, Baudhuin JE, Hullar TE, Washington University Cochlear Implant Study Group. Short-term risk of falling after cochlear implantation. Audiol Neurootol 2014;19(6):370–7.

126. Zur O, Ben-Rubi Shimron H, Leisman G, et al. Balance versus hearing after cochlear implant in an adult. BMJ Case Rep 2017;2017 [pii:bcr-2017-220391].

127. Boisvert I, McMahon CM, Dowell RC. Speech recognition outcomes following bilateral cochlear implantation in adults aged over 50 years old. Int J Audiol 2016;55(Suppl 2):S39–44.

128. Trinidade A, Page JC, Kennett SW, et al. Simultaneous versus sequential bilateral cochlear implants in adults: cost analysis in a US setting. Laryngoscope 2017;127(11):2615–8.

129. van Zon A, Smulders YE, Ramakers GG, et al. Effect of unilateral and simultaneous bilateral cochlear implantation on tinnitus: a prospective study. Laryngoscope 2016;126(4):956–61.

130. Purdy SC, Kelly AS. Change in speech perception and auditory evoked potentials over time after unilateral cochlear implantation in postlingually deaf adults. Semin Hear 2016;37(1):62–73.

131. Távora-Vieira D, De Ceulaer G, Govaerts PJ, et al. Cochlear implantation improves localization ability in patients with unilateral deafness. Ear Hear 2015; 36(3):e93–8.

132. Mertens G, De Bodt M, Van de Heyning P. evaluation of long-term cochlear implant use in subjects with acquired unilateral profound hearing loss: focus on binaural auditory outcomes. Ear Hear 2017;38(1):117–25.

133. Hassepass F, Stabenau V, Arndt S, et al. Magnet dislocation: an increasing and serious complication following MRI in patients with cochlear implants. Rofo 2014;186(7):680–5.

134. Todt I, Tittel A, Ernst A, et al. Pain free 3 T MRI scans in cochlear implantees. Otol Neurotol 2017;38(10):e401–4.

135. Zhang J, Wei W, Ding J, et al. Inroads toward robot-assisted cochlear implant surgery using steerable electrode arrays. Otol Neurotol 2010;31(8):1199–206.

136. Venail F, Bell B, Akkari M, et al. Manual electrode array insertion through a robot-assisted minimal invasive cochleostomy: feasibility and comparison of two different electrode array subtypes. Otol Neurotol 2015;36(6):1015–22.

137. Astolfi L, Simoni E, Giarbini N, et al. Cochlear implant and inflammation reaction: safety study of a new steroid-eluting electrode. Hear Res 2016;336:44–52.

138. Winter JO, Cogan SF, Rizzo JF. Neurotrophin-eluting hydrogel coatings for neural stimulating electrodes. J Biomed Mater Res B Appl Biomater 2007;81(2): 551–63.

139. Richardson RT, Wise AK, Thompson BC, et al. Polypyrrole-coated electrodes for the delivery of charge and neurotrophins to cochlear neurons. Biomaterials 2009;30(13):2614–24.

140. Von Ilberg C, Kiefer J, Tillein J, et al. Electric-acoustic stimulation of the auditory system: new technology for severe hearing loss. ORL J Otorhinolaryngol Relat Spec 1999;61:334–40.

141. Gstoettner WK, Van de Heyning P, O'Connor AF, et al. Electric acoustic stimulation of the auditory system: results of a multicentre investigation. Acta Otolaryngol 2008;12:1–8.

142. Santa Maria PL, Domville-Lewis C, Sucher CM, et al. Hearing preservation surgery for cochlear implantation–hearing and quality of life after 2 years. Otol Neurotol 2013;34(3):526–31.

143. Santa Maria PL, Gluth MB, Yuan Y, et al. Hearing preservation surgery for cochlear implantation: a meta-analysis. Otol Neurotol 2014 Dec;35(10):e256–69.

144. Chen LC, Puschmann S, Debener S. Increased cross-modal functional connectivity in cochlear implant users. Sci Rep 2017;7(1):10043.

145. Cullington H, Kitterick P, DeBold L, et al. Have cochlear implant, won't have to travel: introducing telemedicine to people using cochlear implants. Am J Audiol 2016;25(3S):299–302.

146. Domville-Lewis C, Santa Maria PL, Upson G, et al. Psychophysical map stability in bilateral sequential cochlear implantation: comparing current audiology methods to a new statistical definition. Ear Hear 2015;36(5):497–504.

147. Fujimoto C, Yamasoba T. Oxidative stresses and mitochondrial dysfunction in age-related hearing loss. Oxid Med Cell Longev 2014;2014:582849.

148. Tavanai E, Mohammadkhani G. Role of antioxidants in prevention of age related hearing loss: a review of literature. Eur Arch Otorhinolaryngol 2017;274: 1821–34.

149. Sang L, Zheng T, Min L, et al. Otoprotective effects of ethosuximide in NOD/LtJ mice with age-related hearing loss. Int J Mol Med 2017;40(1):146–54.

150. Syka J, Ouda L, Nachtigal P, et al. Atorvastatin slows down the deterioration of inner ear function with age in mice. Neurosci Lett 2007;411(2):112–6.

151. Mikuriya T, Sugahara K, Sugimoto K, et al. Attenuation of progressive hearing loss in a model of age-related hearing loss by a heat shock protein inducer, geranylgeranylacetone. Brain Res 2008;1212:9–17.

152. Alvardo JC, Fuentes-Santamaria V, Melgar-Rojas P, et al. Synergistic effect of free radical scavengers and cochlear vasodilators: a new otoprotective strategy for age related hearing loss. Front Aging Neurosci 2015;7:86.

153. Chen GD, Kermany MH, D'Elia A, et al. Too much of a good thing: long-term treatment with salicylate strengthens outer hair cell function but impairs auditory neural activity. Hear Res 2010;265(1–2):63–9.

154. Jacob S, Pienkowski M, Fridberger A. The endocochlear potential alters cochlear micromechanics. Biophys J 2011;100(11):2586–94.

155. Someya S, Tanokura M, Weindruch R, et al. Effects of caloric restriction on age-related hearing loss in rodents and rhesus monkeys. Curr Aging Sci 2010;3(1): 20–5.

156. Prehn K, Jumpertz von Schwartzenberg R, Mai K, et al. caloric restriction in older adults-differential effects of weight loss and reduced weight on brain structure and function. Cereb Cortex 2017;27(3):1765–78.

157. Omotehara Y, Hakuba N, Hato N, et al. Protection against ischemic cochlear damage by intratympanic administration of AM-111. Otol Neurotol 2011;32(9): 1422–7.

158. Suckfuell M, Lisowska G, Domka W, et al. Efficacy and safety of AM-111 in the treatment of acute sensorineural hearing loss: a double-blind, randomized, placebo-controlled phase II study. Otol Neurotol 2014;35(8):1317–26.

159. Rubel EW, Furrer SA, Stone JS. A brief history of hair cell regeneration research and speculations on the future. Hear Res 2013;297:42–51.

160. Oshima K, Suchert S, Blevins NH, et al. Curing hearing loss: patient expectations, health care practitioners, and basic science. J Commun Disord 2010; 43(4):311–8.

161. Ronaghi M, Nasr M, Heller S. Concise review: inner ear stem cells–an oxymoron, but why? Stem Cells 2012;30(1):69–74.

162. Mittal R, Nguyen D, Patel AP, et al. Recent advancements in the regeneration of auditory hair cells and hearing restoration. Front Mol Neurosci 2017;10:236.

163. Chow CL, Gubbels SP. Regenerative therapies for sensorineural hearing loss: current research implications for future treatments. In: Sataloff RT, Johns MM, Kost KM, editors. Geriatr Otolaryngology. 2015. p. 63–76.

164. Ahmed H, Shubina-Oleinik O, Holt JR. Emerging gene therapies for genetic hearing loss. J Assoc Res Otolaryngol 2017;18:649–70.

165. Tandon V, Kang WS, Robbins TA, et al. Microfabricated reciprocating micropump for intracochlear drug delivery with integrated drug/fluid storage and electronically controlled dosing. Lab Chip 2016;16(5):829–46.
166. Nieman CL, Lin FR. Increasing access to hearing rehabilitation for older adults. Curr Opin Otolaryngol Head Neck Surg 2017;25(5):342–6.

Vertigo and Dizziness
Understanding and Managing Fall Risk

Jennifer C. Alyono, MD, MS

KEYWORDS

• Vertigo • Dizziness • Fall risk • Geriatric vestibulopathy

KEY POINTS

- Dizziness is associated with functional disability and risk of falls.
- Falls are the leading cause of fatal and nonfatal injuries among older Americans.
- "Dizziness" can describe several sensations, including spinning or nonspinning vertigo, disequilibrium, imbalance, presyncope, lightheadedness, and floating or a combination thereof.
- Chronic dizziness is often multifactorial and can reflect dysfunction in the vestibular, somatosensory, or visual systems or in their central integration. Systemic processes, such as postural hypotension, arrhythmias, heart failure, medication use, and lower extremity weakness or frailty, also contribute.
- Careful history and physical examination are critical in evaluating dizzy patients and in many cases may preclude the need for more expensive imaging or vestibular testing.

INTRODUCTION

Vertigo and dizziness are common among older adults, defined as those over age 65 years. These symptoms are closely associated with fall risk and portend major implications for geriatric injury and disability. Management can be particularly challenging, because symptoms are often nonspecific and may reflect multiple etiologies. This article reviews relevant definitions, epidemiology, pathophysiology of balance, diagnosis, and clinical management.

DEFINITIONS

Dizziness is a general term that can describe several sensations, including spinning or nonspinning vertigo, disequilibrium, presyncope, lightheadedness, floating, or a combination thereof.

- Vertigo refers to the illusory sensation of movement of the body or the environment.

Disclosure: The author has nothing to disclose.
Department of Otolaryngology–Head and Neck Surgery, Stanford University, 801 Welch Road, Stanford, CA 94305, USA
E-mail address: jalyono@stanford.edu

Otolaryngol Clin N Am 51 (2018) 725–740
https://doi.org/10.1016/j.otc.2018.03.003
0030-6665/18/© 2018 Elsevier Inc. All rights reserved.

oto.theclinics.com

- Disequilibrium describes a sense of imbalance, unsteadiness, or postural instability.
- Presyncope connotes lightheadedness and the sense of an impending fainting episode. It is often associated with temporary diffuse cerebral hypoperfusion.

Despite current consensus among medical practitioners as to the use of these terms, patients use these words to describe any or all of the sensations described previously and may also include other sensations, such as weakness, fatigue, floating, fear of falling, or unstable gaze. This discrepancy underlies the importance of asking patients to describe their symptoms in their own words.

EPIDEMIOLOGY

Prevalence studies of dizziness among older adults vary depending on the definition of dizziness, study population (eg, age range or community-dwelling adults vs nursing home), and study setting (eg, emergency department vs primary care). Estimates range from 10% to 35%,[1–4] with rates increasing with age such that up to 50% of community-dwelling adults older than 80 are affected.[5]

Falls are highly associated with vertigo and dizziness.[6] Every 11 seconds, an older adult presents to an emergency room for a fall, and every 19 minutes, an older adult dies from a fall.[7] Even in the absence of falls, dizziness is detrimental to quality of life.[8] Adverse effects include anxiety, decline in mobility, fear of falling, limitations of activities of everyday life, and an increase in indirect health care costs.[8]

PATHOPHYSIOLOGY OF DIZZINESS

Balance involves the central integration of multiple sensory systems: vestibular, vision, and somatosensory proprioception and exteroception. It also involves neuromuscular reflex pathways and core and lower body strength to maintain postural stability in response to perceived stimuli. Dizziness can reflect specific medical conditions affecting single systems or may represent multisensory dysfunction from multiple etiologies (**Table 1**).

The peripheral vestibular system provides information about linear and angular acceleration. Three sets of paired semicircular canals sense angular acceleration. The utricle and saccule (otolithic organs) sense horizontal and vertical linear acceleration, respectively. The canals and otolithic organs are innervated by the vestibular nerve, which projects to the brainstem vestibular nuclei and cerebellum. Efferent tracts from the cerebellum then project to motor nuclei of the extraocular muscles and vestibulospinal tracts, which contribute to gaze stabilization and postural control.

Age-related vestibular loss manifests in decreased vestibular hair cells, fewer vestibular nerve fibers, and loss of cerebellar Purkinje cells. Although older adults consistently show decreased vestibular function on quantitative testing, the presence of dizziness is highly variable: those with objective dysfunction may have no subjective symptoms.[9]

The somatosensory system provides information about proprioception (internal sense of body/limb position) and exteroception (sensation of the environment) from mechanoreceptors in the joints and skin. Information must be relayed through peripheral nerves and the posterior spinal column to reach the central nervous system. In an elevator, the vestibular system's saccule detects vertical acceleration, but mechanoreceptors in the feet simultaneously sense a drop in pressure when going down, and an increase when going up. Common disorders affecting the somatosensory system include arthritis, joint replacements, and peripheral neuropathy from diabetes or vitamin deficiency.

Table 1
Causes of and contributors to dizziness in the elderly

Peripheral vestibular	BPPV
	Vestibular neuritis
	Labyrinthitis
	Late-onset Meniere's disease
	Bilateral deafferentation
	Perilymphatic fistula
	Vestibular schwannoma
Central nervous system	Stroke or transient ischemic attack
	Vertebrobasilar insufficiency
	Vestibular migraine
	Neoplastic
	Neurodegenerative disease (Parkinson's disease, cerebellar ataxia, degenerative dementias)
	(Normal pressure) hydrocephalus
	Multiple sclerosis
	Posttraumatic
	Neurosyphilis
Somatosensory	Peripheral neuropathy (diabetes, vitamin deficiency)
	Cervicogenic vertigo
	Arthritis
Vision	Cataracts
	Use of bifocals/multifocals
Cardiovascular and orthostatic	Arrhythmia
	Heart failure
	Postural hypotension
	Postprandial hypotension
	Hypovolemia
Other systemic	Alcohol
	Heavy metal exposure
	Hypothyroidism
	Hypoglycemia, metabolic imbalance
	Medications, polypharmacy
	Psychophysiologic

Vision provides information about spatial orientation. Visual acuity, depth perception, accommodation, and contrast sensitivity worsen with age. Furthermore, pathologies, such as cataracts and macular degeneration, become more frequent.

Appropriate central integration of sensory information is integral to balance. The brainstem, cerebellum, and higher cortical structures all undergo age-related changes. Neurodegenerative diseases, such as Parkinson's disease and Alzheimer's disease, become more prevalent with age. Stroke, multiple sclerosis, and neoplasias are also possible.

Although the cardiovascular system is not traditionally believed to be directly involved with balance, disorders, such as arrhythmias and orthostatic hypotension, can lead to cerebral hypoperfusion and presyncopal dizziness. Vertebrobasilar insufficiency reflects ischemia of the brain's posterior circulation. Symptoms include vision changes, vertigo, ataxia, and bilateral numbness or weakness. Insufficiency can occur during episodes of reduced blood pressure or flow (such as after periods of standing, hypovolemia, or external vessel compression from neck turn). Other etiologies include atherosclerosis, embolic events, or arterial dissection.

Psychological disease, such as anxiety and depression in particular, are risk factors. They may reflect a psychogenic etiology for dizziness or a psychological response to somatic disease.[10] Other systemic changes, such as electrolyte imbalance, anemia, or hypothyroidism, can lead to fatigue or confusion, which can exacerbate dizziness.

Just as studies of dizziness prevalence vary depending on definitions, population, and setting, studies of etiologies also vary. The most consistent finding is that a majority of patients have multifactorial disease[1,11] (see **Table 1**). Maarsingh and colleagues[1] found that among patients ages 65 to 95 presenting to primary care, cardiovascular (including cerebrovascular) disease represented 57% of all main causes and peripheral otogenic vestibular disease, 14%. Colledge and colleagues[11] studied community-dwelling adults greater than age 65 years and similarly found 70% of persistent dizziness to be caused by "central vascular disease." In contrast, in a younger population with average age 63, Kroenke and colleagues[12] found the peripheral vestibular system the cause in a majority of patients, and benign paroxysmal positional vertigo (BPPV) represented the most common specific etiology.

ADDITIONAL SPECIFIC ETIOLOGIES OF DIZZINESS

Although multisystem and cardiovascular etiologies are the most common causes of dizziness in the elderly, other specific etiologies that are amenable to intervention, such as BPPV, episodic hypotension, and medication-related dizziness, are reviewed.

Benign Paroxysmal Positional Vertigo

Older adults are at increased risk for BPPV, have a higher rate of recurrence, and may report atypical symptoms. BPPV arises from the abnormal displacement of otoconia into the semicircular canals from the saccule or utricle. In canalithiasis, loose debris produces abnormal movement in the endolymph of the canal. In the much rarer cupulolithiasis, debris attaches to the cupula of one of the canals. The posterior canal is most commonly affected, with the lateral canal second.

Most cases of BPPV can be diagnosed using history and provocative maneuvers. A typical patient describes an episodic rotational vertigo lasting less than a minute, provoked when changing head position relative to gravity, such as turning over in bed.

Physicians should perform the Dix-Hallpike maneuver for further evaluation (discussed later; **Fig. 1**). In cases where history suggests BPPV but the Dix-Hallpike maneuver is negative, the supine roll test can be performed to assess for lateral canal BPPV. At presentation, multiple canals may be involved, and treatment of posterior canal BPPV can lead to otoconia being displaced into the lateral canal. The American Academy of Otolaryngology–Head and Neck Surgery recommends that patients who meet criteria for BPPV without inconsistent signs/symptoms should not obtain routine imaging or vestibular testing.

Episodic Hypotension

Patients with orthostatic hypotension present with dizziness on standing or sitting up. Orthostatic hypotension is defined as a decrease in systolic blood pressure by 20 mm Hg or in diastolic blood pressure by 10 mm Hg within 3 minutes of standing. Hypovolemia, vasodilation, and disorders of the cardiovascular, neurologic, or endocrine systems can be causative.

In the elderly, postprandial hypotension is another consideration. It is characterized by systolic blood pressure decrease by 20 mm Hg or fall below 90 mm Hg within

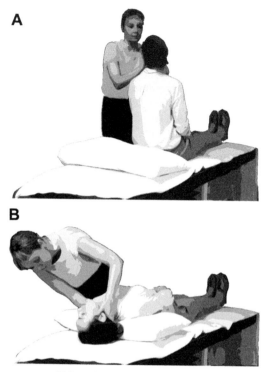

Fig. 1. Dix-Hallpike maneuver. This patient is being assessed for left posterior canal BPPV. (*A*) The examiner stands beside the patient, whose head is turned 45° to the left. (*B*) The patient is guided from seated to supine, with neck extended. Neck extension is achieved by allowing the patient's head to extend beyond the end of the table or by placing a cushion under the shoulders. The patient keeps her eyes open, allowing the physician to examine for nystagmus. After nystagmus resolves, or after 30 seconds, the patient is guided back to a seated position. (*Courtesy of* Jennifer C. Alyono, MD, MS, Stanford, CA.)

2 hours after meals.[13] It is believed to result from a deficient sympathetic response after eating.[13] Treatment includes increasing preprandial water intake, decreasing carbohydrates, and eating more frequent, smaller meals.

Medication-Related Dizziness

Many drugs can cause or exacerbate dizziness (**Box 1**). This is particularly troublesome in the elderly, who have reduced hepatic and renal clearance of drugs, and may have increased sensitivity to drugs. Dizziness can be potentiated through numerous mechanisms: direct ototoxicity, lowering of blood pressure, volume depletion, or direct central nervous system depression and sedation.

DIAGNOSTIC APPROACH TO PATIENTS WITH DIZZINESS

Evaluation of patients with dizziness can be challenging for both patients and physicians alike—symptoms can be difficult to describe and potential diagnoses broad. Although a single cause is not always identifiable, addressing contributors to dysfunction can alleviate, if not resolve, dizziness symptoms in addition to reducing the risk of fall.

Box 1
Medications that may cause dizziness

Ototoxic—peripheral vestibular impairment
   Aminoglycosides
   Loop diuretics
   Platinum-based and vinca alkaloid chemotherapeutics

Cardiovascular—hypotension
   β-blockers and calcium channel blockers
   Vasodilators
   Diuretics
   Angiotensin-converting enzyme inhibitors, angiotensin II receptor blockers

Psychoactive
   Benzodiazepines
   Barbiturates
   Benzodiazepine receptor agonists (eg, zolpidem, zopiclone, and zaleplon)
   Anticonvulsants
   Antidepressants
   Opioids
   Antipsychotics

Antihistamines

Anticholinergics

Muscle relaxants

History

A detailed history is invaluable. Patients should describe their dizziness in their own words. Physicians should inquire about the duration and intensity of symptoms, whether dizziness is constant or episodic, and the length of specific episodes, if applicable. Precipitating factors (such as meals and certain movements) and associated symptoms (such as hearing loss, vision changes, headache, palpitations, chest pain, numbness, and weakness) should be elicited. Recent events, such as trauma and bleeding, may be relevant.

A full medication history should be taken, including over-the-counter drugs, supplements, recreational drugs, and alcohol. A complete medical history should be asked for, with particular attention to disorders that may contribute to fall risk, including cardiovascular disease, arrhythmias, ophthalmologic disease, anemia, arthritis, diabetes, depression, or anxiety.

Physical

Physical examination should be thorough but also focused on the neurologic system. Screening for orthostatic hypotension is recommended as part of routine vital signs. Pulse palpation and heart auscultation can reveal arrhythmias.

Examination of the ears should assess for otitis media or middle ear effusion. Finger rub and tuning fork tests can screen for asymmetric hearing loss.

A complete cranial nerve examination is recommended. On assessing extraocular movements, observe for spontaneous or gaze-evoked nystagmus (**Table 2**). The extremities should be evaluated for sensation and strength. Cogwheeling may suggest Parkinson's disease.

The Romberg test assesses the vestibular and proprioceptive systems. A patient is asked to stand with eyes closed and feet next to each other. The sharpened Romberg is more challenging, with a patient asked to stand with 1 foot in front of the other, in

Table 2
Peripheral versus central oculomotor abnormalities

	Peripheral	Central
Gaze-evoked nystagmus	Unidirectional	Direction may change with gaze position
Spontaneous nystagmus	Horizontal and/or torsional; suppressed by gaze fixation	Often pure vertical, horizontal, or torsional; not suppressed by gaze fixation
Head impulse test	Impaired	Intact
Provocative positional testing (ie Dix-Hallpike maneuver)	Longer latency; fatigability present	Shorter or absent latency; no fatigability present
Smooth pursuit	Smooth	Catch-up saccades

tandem. Regular gait and tandem gait are assessed. A cerebellar examination also includes assessment for dysdiadochokinesia, using rapid alternating hand movements, and for dysmetria, using the finger to nose test.

Provocative Maneuvers

Provocative maneuvers can further assess the vestibular system.

The Dix-Hallpike maneuver is used to evaluate for posterior canal BPPV (see **Fig. 1**). Three key features should be observed to confirm the diagnosis of posterior canal BPPV:

- Nystagmus is torsional and upbeating.
- There is a latency period of approximately 5 seconds to 20 seconds between maneuver completion and onset of subjective vertigo and objective nystagmus.
- The vertigo and nystagmus crescendo and then decrescendo, resolving within 60 seconds.

In the head impulse test (also known as head thrust test) (**Fig. 2**), the examiner sits face-to-face with the patient, with head upright. The patient fixes the gaze on a target (such as the examiner's nose). The examiner rapidly rotates the patient's head left or right or back to midline while observing for corrective saccades. A corrective saccade (where the eyes initially follow the head movement before saccading back to the target) indicates an abnormal test, reflective of vestibular disease. The test is abnormal when the head is thrust toward the side of vestibulopathy. For example, a patient with left vestibular neuritis has corrective saccades when the head is thrust to the left.

In the test of skew (also known as alternate cover test), the examiner covers 1 eye, then the other, switching back and forth. In a healthy patient, the eyes remain motionless. The test is positive, or abnormal, when the eye has a refixation saccade after the cover is moved, indicating ocular misalignment. A positive test can reflect longstanding strabismus; on the other hand, in an acutely vertiginous patient, vertical ocular misalignment strongly suggests posterior fossa stroke.

STUDIES
Laboratory

No consensus exists on standardized laboratory tests. Instead, testing should be tailored to a patient's specific situation. For example, a patient meeting diagnostic criteria for BPPV may need no further testing. In contrast, a patient with acute

Normal: Eyes remain looking at examiner with head thrust, reflecting intact vestibulo-ocular reflex.

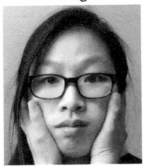
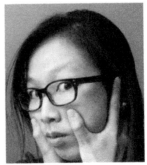

Right vestibulopathy: Corrective saccade observed after head is thrust toward the affected side.

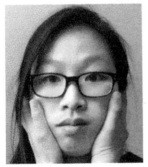
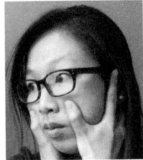
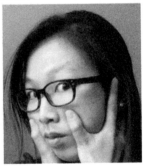

Fig. 2. Head impulse test.

dizziness and chest pain warrants cardiac enzymes. In chronic multifactorial dizziness, hematocrit, basic metabolic panel, hemoglobin A_{1C}, and vitamin B_{12} levels may help rule out systemic contributors.

Audiometry

Many patients with age-related loss of vestibular function also have age-related hearing loss. In corollary, insults to the vestibular system (Meniere's disease and ototoxic medications) are also likely to affect hearing. Screening for hearing loss is recommended, because hearing loss is an additional risk factor for social isolation, depression, and cognitive decline.

Vestibular Testing

Often, careful history and physical examination are sufficient for diagnosis and management of dizziness. In some cases, judicious use of specialized vestibular testing is helpful (**Table 3**). Formal vestibular testing is indicated when the side or site of pathology cannot be localized by history and physical, in documentation of contralateral function when vestibular ablation in considered, and at times, when tracking disease progression or recovery.

Table 3
Vestibular testing

Assessment	Description	System Tested	Clinical Utility
Electronystagmography or videonystagmography			
Eye movements are quantitatively recorded in these subtests:			
Oculomotor	Smooth pursuit, saccadic, and optokinetic tracking	Central and peripheral vestibular	May distinguish central vs peripheral etiology (see **Table 2**)
Spontaneous and static positional nystagmus	Sitting, supine, body right/left, head turned, etc.		
Caloric testing	Irrigate ear canal with 30°C cool and/or 44°C warm water	Horizontal semicircular canals	Quantifies relative weakness of left vs right.
Dix-Hallpike maneuver	See **Fig. 1** for maneuver description	Canalithiasis or cupulolithaisis	Helpful when clinical Dix-Hallpike maneuver is equivocal or atypical
Rotational chair	Compares eye movement responses to head/ body rotation.	Vestibulo-ocular reflex	Only test that can detect bilateral vestibular deficits
VEMPs			
Cervical VEMP	Surface electrodes record the sternocleidomastoid (cervical VEMP) or the inferior oblique eye muscles (ocular VEMP) in response to sound stimuli	Saccule, inferior vestbular nerve, vestibulocolic reflex	Diagnostic for superior semicircular canal dehiscence Unreliable if conductive hearing loss present
Ocular VEMP		Utricle, superior vestibular nerve	
Head impulse test with video-oculography	Eye movements are recorded while the head is thrust multidirectionally. Accelerometers record head velocity and direction.	Semicircular canals, vestibulo-ocular reflex	High-frequency, high-acceleration test of the semicircular canals
Computerized dynamic posturography			
Sensory organization test	Ability to maintain balance with eyes open vs closed, with stable vs moving platform, with or without visual surround discordant to sway	Assesses ability to use vestibular vs visual vs proprioceptive systems to maintain balance	Guides and tracks progress to vestibular therapy. Can also use in cases of suspected malingering.

Abbreviation: VEMP, vestibular-evoked myogenic potentials.

Imaging

Many investigators agree that routine neuroimaging is unlikely to reveal the cause of dizziness in most patients.[14,15] Often, imaging findings are present, such as cortical atrophy, but do not alter management, thus requiring nuanced interpretation.[14]

Commonly accepted indications for neuroimaging include focal neurologic signs, suspicion for acute stroke, asymmetric symptoms (such as unilateral hearing loss), known vascular abnormalities, or recent trauma. CT is superior in demonstrating bony abnormalities (eg, superior semicircular canal dehiscence), whereas MRI is superior in demonstrating soft tissue.

ACUTE VESTIBULAR SYNDROME

Special mention is warranted in assessing acute vestibular syndrome (AVS). Acute unilateral injury to the peripheral or central vestibular system produces AVS and is manifested by continuous vertigo, nausea/vomiting, nystagmus, and motion intolerance that evolve over the course of hours.[16,17] Although vestibular neuritis is a common etiology and is self-limited with good long-term prognosis, stroke involving the posterior circulation can present similarly but with potentially more devastating consequences. For example, edema from inferior cerebellar stroke can lead to brainstem compression and death.[16] Misdiagnosis of stroke occurs far more frequently in those presenting with dizziness (35%) compared with those with motor deficits (4%).[18]

Acute vertigo from brainstem stroke is often but not always accompanied by additional symptoms, such as diplopia, dysarthria, other cranial neuropathies, or focal sensory or motor deficits.[16] One study found that up to three-fourths of patients with posterior circulation stroke had isolated AVS with no other symptoms.[17] Dysmetria, pathognomonic for cerebellar dysfunction, may be minimal or even absent after inferior cerebellar stroke.[16] Patients with acute unilateral peripheral vestibulopathy often fall toward the affected side but are typically able to ambulate. In contrast, those with acute cerebellar stroke are usually unable to walk.[16]

The HINTS "plus" battery is a useful three-step bedside examination for patients with AVS. HINTS stands for Head Impulse, Nystagmus, and Test of Skew (see **Table 4**). Compared with early MRI, which can be falsely negative in half of patients up to 48 hours after symptom onset, HINTS "plus" is highly accurate, with a sensitivity of 98%, specificity of 85%, and negative likelihood ratio of 2%.[17,19]

Stroke should be suspected if any one of the following is true: the head impulse test is normal (see **Fig. 2**), nystagmus is direction-changing or vertical (see **Table 3**), or skew deviation (ocular misalignment) is present on the alternate cover test. Conversely, a patient with peripheral vertigo should have an abnormal head impulse test, unidirectional non-vertical nystagmus, and no skew deviation.

HINTS "plus" includes acute hearing loss (in the absence of middle ear disease) as a sign of anterior inferior cerebellar artery infarction. Although including hearing loss in this battery decreases specificity, it increases sensitivity, and therefore decreases the risk of missed stroke. Contrary to conventional teaching, recent studies suggest

Table 4	
H.I.N.T.S. examination for acute vestibular syndrome	
Examination Steps: H.I.N.T.S.	**Findings in Stroke: I.N.F.A.R.C.T.**
Head *I*mpulse test (head thrust)	*I*mpulse *N*ormal
*N*ystagmus	*F*ast-phase *A*lternating (direction changes with gaze or vertical)
*T*est of *S*kew (alternate cover test)	*R*efixation on *C*over *T*est (skew deviation present)

Adapted from Newman-Toker DE, Kerber KA, Hsieh YH, et al. HINTS outperforms ABCD2 to screen for stroke in acute continuous vertigo and dizziness. Acad Emerg Med 2013;20(10):988; with permission.

that the presence of associated acute hearing loss more often reflects vascular infarction rather than viral labyrinthis.[20]

A neurologist should be consulted early should stroke be suspected.

MANAGEMENT OF PATIENTS WITH DIZZINESS

Disease-directed therapy should be initiated in cases with specific diagnoses, such as BPPV. In the absence of focal diagnosis, treatment consists of reducing symptoms, managing risk factors, and reducing fall risk.

Medications

Drugs commonly used as vestibular suppressants include antihistamines (eg, meclizine and diphenhydramine), anticholinergics (eg, scopolamine), antidopaminergics (eg, metoclopramide), benzodiazepines (eg, diazepam and clonazepam), and phenothiazines (eg, promethazine and prochlorperazine, which have antidopaminergic, antihistaminergic, and anticholinergic properties). These medications may be useful in the acute setting for

- Relief of nausea/vomiting in acute vertigo
- Prevention of nausea prior to planned canalith repositioning maneuvers in BPPV
- Prevention of motion sickness

None, however, is appropriate for long-term use in chronic dizziness, and many investigators recommend discontinuation after 3 days.[21] Vestibular suppressants compromise physiologic compensation, prolonging symptoms of dizziness, and may lead to dependency. Side effects are particularly troubling in the elderly and include delirium, cognitive impairment, and urinary retention.

Certain pharmaceuticals are indicated for specific pathologies:

- Vestibular neuronitis/labyrinthitis: steroids have been shown to decrease acute symptom length and improve long-term recovery of vestibular function.
- Vestibular migraine: prophylactic β-blockers, calcium channel blockers, anticonvulsants, and antidepressants
- Meniere's disease: prophylactic diuretics; for exacerbations: intratympanic or systemic steroids, intratympanic gentamycin for ablation

Canalith Repositioning Maneuvers for Benign Paroxysmal Positional Vertigo

The mainstay of BPPV treatment is canalith repositioning maneuvers, such as the Epley or Semont maneuvers. Brandt-Daroff maneuvers are exercises patients perform at home and are intended to catalyze compensation and habituation.

The Epley begins similarly to a Dix-Hallpike test (**Fig. 3**):

- Starting seated with the head turned toward the symptomatic side (for example, the right), the patient is laid back to supine with the head gently extended.
- The patient's head is then rotated 90° toward the opposite, left side.
- Next, the patient continues rotating the head to the left, by looking down toward the ground as he or she rolls onto the left shoulder, into lateral decubitus position.
- In the final step, the patient then is sat upright.
- Each position is maintained for 20 seconds to 30 seconds, allowing vertigo to resolve.

Additional detail regarding the Semont maneuver, treatment of cupulolithais, and disease affecting the lateral canal can be found in the American Academy of Otolaryngology–Head and Neck Surgery clinical practice guidelines.[22]

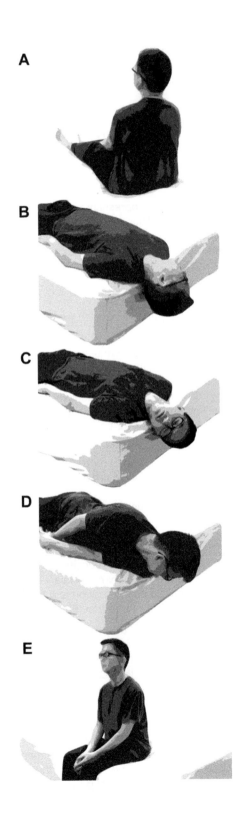

Vestibular Therapy

Vestibular rehabilitation not only is useful in reducing falls but also helpful in decreasing dizziness symptoms, regardless of etiology. Vestibular therapy catalyzes compensation in 3 ways[23]:

- Adaptation (central gain readjustment in vestibulospinal or vestibulo-ocular reflexes)
- Substitution (strengthening nonvestibular components of balance)
- Habituation (reducing maladaptive responses and increasing sensory thresholds through repetitive exposure to provocative situations)

Fall Risk Assessment

In addition to treating patients' symptoms of vertigo and dizziness, directed assessments of fall risk should be made. The American Geriatrics Society and British Geriatrics Society published a joint recommendation for annual multifactorial fall risk assessment in all adults over 65 years.[24] Patients are considered high risk if they answer yes to any of the following:

1. Two or more falls in the past 12 months?
2. Presenting with an acute fall?
3. Difficulty with walking or balance?

Given the widespread impact of falls, multiple national and international organizations have outlined algorithms for fall risk assessment and reduction.[7,24] The Centers for Disease Control and Prevention Stopping Elderly Accidents, Deaths, and Injuries (STEADI) toolkit is a good example (https://www.cdc.gov/steadi/).

Patients who screen positive can then be assessed for gait, strength, and balance using standardized tests, such as the Timed Up and Go, 30-Second Chair Stand, or 4-Stage Balance Test. Additional assessment includes history of postural hypotension, medication review, feet and footwear examination, and vision assessment. Dementia is another important consideration, because its presence not only impairs balance but also decreases hazard recognition.

Fall Risk Reduction

Once patients have been identified as high risk for falls, multifactorial intervention should be implemented.

Medication minimization

Polypharmacy, especially psychotropic medication, has consistently been associated with falls. If discontinuation of medications is not possible, dose reduction should be considered.

Exercise programs

In addition to formal vestibular therapy, home-based and community exercise programs[25] (such as tai chi) that emphasize strength and balance are effective.

◀─────────────────────────────

Fig. 3. Epley maneuver. This patient is being treated for right posterior canal BPPV. (*A*) The patient starts seated, then (*B*) is laid supine with head turned to the symptomatic side (*right*) and neck extended. (*C*) The patient's head is then rotated 90° to the opposite side (*left*). (*D*) The patient continues rotating the head to the left, looking down toward the ground as he rolls onto his left shoulder, into lateral decubitus position. (*E*) In the final step, the patient is sat upright. Each position is maintained for 20 seconds to 30 seconds, allowing vertigo to resolve.

Assistive devices
A physical therapist can determine whether a patient would benefit from a mobility aid, such as a cane or walker.

Vision impairment
Cataract surgery has shown the most effectiveness in reducing falls.[24] Importantly, patients should avoid multifocal or bifocal lenses while walking, especially on stairs. Bifocals distort depth perception, making tripping accidents more likely.

Vitamin D
The American Geriatrics Society instructs that vitamin D should be recommended in all patients with deficiency and considered in those otherwise at high fall risk.[24] Vitamin D supplementation is believed not only to reduce falls by improving neuromuscular function but also to decrease fracture risk in the event of a fall.[26]

Foot and footwear intervention
Bunions or toe deformities may require podiatry consultation. Footwear choices are also important: shoes with low heel height, high contact area with the ground, and good fit are recommended.

Home modification
Patients should evaluate their surroundings for modifiable hazards:

- Removing trip hazards inside the home, like throw rugs and low-lying furniture
- Removing trip hazards outside the home, such as cracked sidewalks and exposed tree roots
- Improving nighttime illumination
- Installing hand-rails in bathrooms and stairs

SUMMARY

Vertigo and dizziness are common among older adults and are associated with heightened fall risk. Multisensory deficits are common, and multifactorial etiologies may contribute. History and physical examination are integral to diagnosis and may preclude the need for imaging or specialized vestibular testing. In AVS, HINTS is a useful screening battery for stroke. In patients with chronic dizziness, formal fall risk assessment should be performed, and multilimbed interventions implemented. Vestibular therapy is effective in reducing both symptom severity and fall risk.

REFERENCES

1. Maarsingh OR, Stam H, van de Ven PM, et al. Predictors of dizziness in older persons: a 10-year prospective cohort study in the community. BMC Geriatr 2014;14:133.
2. Olsson Moller U, Midlov P, Kristensson J, et al. Prevalence and predictors of falls and dizziness in people younger and older than 80 years of age–a longitudinal cohort study. Arch Gerontol Geriatr 2013;56(1):160–8.
3. Agrawal Y, Carey JP, Della Santina CC, et al. Disorders of balance and vestibular function in US adults: data from the National Health and Nutrition Examination Survey, 2001-2004. Arch Intern Med 2009;169(10):938–44.
4. Lin HW, Bhattacharyya N. Balance disorders in the elderly: epidemiology and functional impact. Laryngoscope 2012;122(8):1858–61.

5. Colledge NR, Wilson JA, Macintyre CC, et al. The prevalence and characteristics of dizziness in an elderly community. Age Ageing 1994;23(2):117–20.

6. Tuunainen E, Rasku J, Jantti P, et al. Risk factors of falls in community dwelling active elderly. Auris Nasus Larynx 2014;41(1):10–6.

7. Fall prevention fact sheet. Arlington (VA): National Council on Aging; 2016. p. 1–2.

8. Dros J, Maarsingh OR, Beem L, et al. Impact of dizziness on everyday life in older primary care patients: a cross-sectional study. Health Qual Life Outcomes 2011; 9:44.

9. Davalos-Bichara M, Agrawal Y. Normative results of healthy older adults on standard clinical vestibular tests. Otol Neurotol 2014;35(2):297–300.

10. Carmeli E. Anxiety in the elderly can be a vestibular problem. Front Public Health 2015;3:216.

11. Colledge NR, Barr-Hamilton RM, Lewis SJ, et al. Evaluation of investigations to diagnose the cause of dizziness in elderly people: a community based controlled study. BMJ 1996;313(7060):788–92.

12. Kroenke K, Lucas CA, Rosenberg ML, et al. Causes of persistent dizziness. A prospective study of 100 patients in ambulatory care. Ann Intern Med 1992; 117(11):898–904.

13. Luciano GL, Brennan MJ, Rothberg MB. Postprandial hypotension. Am J Med 2010;123(3):281.e1-e6.

14. Connor S, Sriskandan N. Imaging of dizziness. Clin Radiol 2013;69(2):111–22.

15. Nanda A, Besdine R. Dizziness [Chapter 50]. In: Halter J, Ouslander J, Studenski S, et al, editors. Hazzard's geriatric medicine and gerontology, 7e. 7th edition. New York: McGraw-Hill Education; 2017.

16. Hotson JR, Baloh RW. Acute vestibular syndrome. N Engl J Med 1998;339(10): 680–5.

17. Saber Tehrani AS, Kattah JC, Mantokoudis G, et al. Small strokes causing severe vertigo: frequency of false-negative MRIs and nonlacunar mechanisms. Neurology 2014;83(2):169–73.

18. Newman-Toker DE, Moy E, Valente E, et al. Missed diagnosis of stroke in the emergency department: a cross-sectional analysis of a large population-based sample. Diagnosis (Berl) 2014;1(2):155–66.

19. Tarnutzer A, Berkowitz A, Robinson K, et al. Does my dizzy patient have a stroke? A systematic review of bedisde diagnosis in acute vestibuar syndrome. Can Med Assoc J 2011;183(9):E571–92.

20. Newman-Toker DE, Kerber KA, Hsieh YH, et al. HINTS outperforms ABCD2 to screen for stroke in acute continuous vertigo and dizziness. Acad Emerg Med 2013;20(10):986–96.

21. Lo AX, Harada CN. Geriatric dizziness: evolving diagnostic and therapeutic approaches for the emergency department. Clin Geriatr Med 2013;29(1):181–204.

22. Bhattacharyya N, Gubbels SP, Schwartz SR, et al. Clinical practice guideline: benign paroxysmal positional vertigo (update). Otolaryngol Head Neck Surg 2017;156(3_suppl):S1–47.

23. Han BI, Song HS, Kim JS. Vestibular rehabilitation therapy: review of indications, mechanisms, and key exercises. J Clin Neurol 2011;7(4):184–96.

24. Panel on Prevention of Falls in Older Persons, American Geriatrics Society and British Geriatrics Society. Summary of the Updated American Geriatrics Society/British Geriatrics Society clinical practice guideline for prevention of falls in older persons. J Am Geriatr Soc 2011;59(1):148–57.

25. Low S, Ang LW, Goh KS, et al. A systematic review of the effectiveness of Tai Chi on fall reduction among the elderly. Arch Gerontol Geriatr 2009;48(3): 325–31.
26. Bischoff-Ferrari HA, Dawson-Hughes B, Staehelin HB, et al. Fall prevention with supplemental and active forms of vitamin D: a meta-analysis of randomised controlled trials. BMJ 2009;339:b3692.

Head and Neck Cancer and the Elderly Patient

Brian P. Cervenka, MD[a,*], Shyam Rao, MD[b], Arnaud F. Bewley, MD[a]

KEYWORDS

- Head and neck cancer • Elderly medicine • Surgical therapy • Radiation therapy
- Chemotherapy • Comprehensive elderly assessment

KEY POINTS

- Surgery, radiation, and chemotherapy have equivalent oncologic efficacy in elderly patients.
- Elderly patients are more likely to suffer from multiple comorbid conditions and decreased functional status.
- Comorbid conditions and decreased functional status increase the risk of treatment-induced morbidity.
- Using screening tools to evaluate comorbid conditions and functional status can help stratify patients, predict treatment toxicity, and guide treatment decisions.
- Elderly patients should be closely observed for toxicity during treatment.

INTRODUCTION

Head and neck cancer is the sixth most prevalent malignancy worldwide.[10] It disproportionately affects older patients, with approximately 50% of new head and neck cancer diagnoses occurring in patients over age 60, and 70% of deaths occurring in patients over age 70.[7] Older age has been shown to be an independent risk factor for head and neck cancer.[11] As the US population continues to age, there will be a higher percentage of patients requiring cancer treatment who are defined as elderly, with elderly defined by the National Institutes of Health National Institute on Aging as any patient 65 years of age or older.[12] It is, therefore, critical that health care providers have an understanding of the nuances of treatment of this disease in the elderly population.

A majority of elderly patients present with stage 3 or stage 4 disease.[3] Although many of these patients would benefit from aggressive, multimodality therapy, their

Disclosure: The authors have nothing to disclose.
[a] Department of Otolaryngology, Division of Head and Neck Surgery, University of California, Davis, 2521 Stockton Boulevard, Sacramento, CA 95817, USA; [b] Department of Radiation Oncology, University of California, Davis, 4501 X Street, Sacramento, CA 95817, USA
* Corresponding author. 2521 Stockton Boulevard, Suite 7200, Sacramento, CA 95817.
E-mail address: bcervenka@ucdavis.edu

Otolaryngol Clin N Am 51 (2018) 741–751
https://doi.org/10.1016/j.otc.2018.03.004
0030-6665/18/© 2018 Elsevier Inc. All rights reserved.

advanced age and higher incidence of medical comorbidities can motivate providers to de-escalate their therapy. Moye and colleagues[5] showed this undertreatment is associated with poorer outcomes. Stage-appropriate multimodality therapy in elderly patients, however, led to equivalent survival outcomes as in younger controls in a large retrospective series. In addition, elderly patients are under-represented in the literature and there are few retrospective data and almost no prospective data to guide treatment modifications for this group of patients.[8] In an attempt to mitigate these challenges, screening tools have been developed to stratify elderly patients into those who would tolerate standard therapy versus those who would be at increased risk for suffering excess toxicity.

This article discusses the oncologic outcomes and risks associated with surgical management, radiation therapy, and chemotherapy in elderly head and neck cancer patients. In addition, currently available screening tools are reviewed and their role in identifying high-risk elderly patients discussed.

SURGERY

Surgery is a common treatment modality for head and neck cancer and is a major determinant of locoregional control and treatment-associated morbidity. Multiple studies have shown that oncologic outcomes after primary surgery are independent of age (**Table 1**).[12–14] Four small retrospective single-institution series have compared survival outcomes for head and neck cancer patients treated with primary surgery between age groups. Three of these showed no difference in the 5-year survival rates between the older and younger groups.[12–14] Clayman and colleagues,[15] however, reported inferior survival in patients over the age of 80 compared with patients under the age of 65 but noted that the survival in the 80 plus group was equivalent to octogenarians without cancer. In 1 of the largest series, Bhattacharyya and colleagues used the Surveillance, Epidemiology, and End Results (SEER) database to compare 2548 surgically managed patients over age 70 with glottic, tongue, or tonsillar squamous cell carcinomas to younger controls. They found that there was a statistically significant decrease in overall survival and disease-specific survival in the glottic and anterior tongue subgroups but not the tonsillar subgroup. This trend was observed when each subgroup was stratified by stage but this was not consistently statistically significant. It is difficult to identify why the elderly group had an overall worse survival given that there is no description of differences in comorbidity or treatment received.

Perioperative Complications

Perioperative complications after primary surgical management of head and neck cancer also seem largely independent of age. There are 5 retrospective series that have shown no increase in postoperative complication rates in elderly patients.[1,12–15] Zabrodsky and colleagues[9] found that advanced-stage disease, comorbidity, and longer operative times were independently associated with increased incidence of complications and found no such association with age. Audisio and colleagues[2] similarly found an association between comorbidity index, as measured by the Adult Comorbidity Evaluation (ACE)-27 or the Charlson Comorbidity Index, and major complications but not age. In a study looking at the 30-day readmission rates after laryngectomy, the elderly group had a higher readmission rate, but this was also correlated to comorbidities, marital status, extent of surgical resection, dysphagia, pneumonia, and cardiovascular complications.[16] Morgan and colleagues[17] did find a higher 30-day mortality rate for older patients in a large retrospective series; however, this

Table 1
Surgical outcomes in geriatric patients undergoing head and neck ablative surgery

Author	Study Type	No. of Patients	Morbidity Outcomes	Survival Outcomes	Summary
Milet et al,[12] 2010	Retrospective single institution	261 patients 29 age 70 and older and 232 <70 y	No significant difference in complications between groups	Risk factors for death on multivariate analysis showed that larynx cancer and female gender are significant, not age >70.	Age 70 or greater not associated with increased risk of death
Zabrodsky et al,[9] 2004	Retrospective single institution	24 patients over age 70	Complication rate 63%, clinically important complication rate 54%	Not assessed	Longer operative times, comorbidity, and advanced stage associated with complication rate
Bhattacharyya et al,[6] 2003	Retrospective SEER study	1882 glottic, 426 oral tongue, 200 tonsillar Patients ages 70 and older (elderly) matched to 5069 controls	Not assessed	Glottic: overall survival 73.9 mo in elderly group vs 96.7 mo in control (P<.05) Oral cavity: overall survival 59.5 mo in elderly and 73.1 mo control (P<.05) Tonsillar: overall survival no significant difference	Overall survival in grouped all stages trend toward decreased overall survival in elderly patients in glottic, oral tongue but not tonsillar When stage stratified, this trend present but not significant in stage 2 glottic, stage 3 and 4 oral tongue, and all tonsillar stages
Blackwell et al,[19] 2002	Retrospective single institution All undergoing microvascular reconstruction	13 patients age 80 or greater	No flap failure Medical complication rate 64% vs 15% in younger controls	Not assessed	Significantly higher rate of medical complications in older group Suggest related to increased comorbidities

(continued on next page)

Table 1
(continued)

Author	Study Type	No. of Patients	Morbidity Outcomes	Survival Outcomes	Summary
					No increase in surgical complications
Clayman et al,[15] 1998	Respective single institution	122 patients, 43 patients age 80 or greater, 79 patients 80 or younger	No significant difference in postoperative complications	Age 80 or greater had a lower overall survival and disease-specific survival (P<.05)	No significant difference in postoperative complications but a significantly lower overall survival in patients >80 y
Shaari et al,[14] 1998	Retrospective single-institution study All undergoing microvascular reconstruction	87 patients, 52 age 70 or older, 35 patients less than age 70	Patients age 70 or older had a complication. Rate of 48% vs 57% in patients younger than 70 (P>.05) Age had no impact on complication rates on multivariate regression.	Patients age 70 or older had a mortality rate of 6% vs 0% in younger than 70. Significance or risk factors not noted	Age did not have an impact on postoperative complications in patients undergoing resection followed by microvascular free flap reconstruction. Mortality rate higher in over-70 age group
McGuirt et al,[1] 1995	Retrospective single institution	217; divided 65–71 y (49), 72–74 y (55), 75–80 y (56), >80 y (57)	Complications (%): 65–71 (19), 72–74 (22), 75–80 (28), >80 (32)	5-y survival: 65–71 (49), 72–74 (55), 75–80 (56), >80 (57)	No significant difference in survival between patients ages >80 and 65–71 No significant difference in complication rates

Bridger et al,[18] 1994	Retrospective single institution All undergoing microvascular reconstruction	117 patients; 26 patients ages 70 and older, 91 under 70 y	42% of patients age 70 and older had postoperative complications vs 37% in patients under 70 (P>.05) Medical complications 54% in ages 70 and older, and 29% in <70 y	Not assessed	No significant difference in postoperative surgical complications or postoperative medical complications in patients with <2 comorbidities Not stated the difference between patients with >2 comorbidities
Kowalski et al,[13] 1994	Retrospective single institution	230 patients, 115 ages 70 or older and 115 younger than age 70	No significant difference in postoperative complications, mortality, or recurrences	5-y survival rate for age 70 or older group was 43% and 55.6% in the control group (P>.05)	No significant difference between patients ages 70 or older and controls in postoperative complications or survival
Morgan et al,[17] 1982	Retrospective single institution	810 patients age 65 or older	Complication rate 32% in patients age 65 or greater and 21% in patients <65	Perioperative mortality (30 d) was 3.5% in elderly group and 0.8% in patients under 65	Significant difference in both survival and complications with the older patients having a higher percentage Not matched based on stage, morbidity, surgery type performed

was in comparison to a cohort that was not matched with respect to stage and comorbidity. Bridger and colleagues[18] found a higher number of complications in elderly patients who had more than 2 preexisting comorbidities compared with younger controls.

Free Flaps

Microvascular free flaps are frequently used to reconstruct head and neck surgical defects. Two retrospective studies have looked at the outcomes of microvascular free flaps in elderly patients and, similar to ablative surgery, concluded that there is not an increased risk of surgical complication. These studies did show an incidence of medical complications in older patients that was also associated with the patient comorbidities.[14,18] Blackwell and colleagues[19] looked at a series of 13 patients over 80 years old and found a higher cost and higher risk of complications even when controlling for comorbidity. They argue that the cost and the higher risk of complications should be carefully considered when undertaking these operations in elderly patients.

Quality of Life

Quality of life is an important consideration after definitive surgical therapy. Khafif and colleagues[4] administered the University of Washington, Quality of Life Questionnaire to patients between ages 65 to 75 and over age 75 who had undergone head and neck surgery and found that older patients tend to score less on several domains of quality of life. They attributed this primarily to a more pronounced effect of pain on their daily activities, an inability to resume normal life due to emotional and physical limitations, and the sense of burden on their caregivers.[4] Dhiwakar and colleagues[20] also found that quality of life decreases after surgical management of head and neck cancer but the change in quality of life was the same for younger and older aged patients.

Elderly patients seem to have largely similar oncologic and perioperative surgical outcomes to younger patients. Perioperative complications have been better associated with comorbidity, extent of surgical resection, and duration of anesthesia time. Therefore, surgical decisions for these patients should weigh patient comorbidity, functional status, social support, and patient goals over age.

RADIATION THERAPY

Radiation therapy is effective in the treatment of head and neck cancer and is used both in the definitive setting and in the adjuvant setting after surgery. Radiation can have many side effects, including mucositis with associated severe pain, xerostomia, skin reaction, fatigue, loss of taste and hypothyroidism. Chronic side effects include osteoradionecrosis, muscle fibrosis, trismus and secondary malignancy. In patients with limited functional status at baseline, these side effects can be debilitating and treatment breaks and significant morbidity seen.

Similar to surgical management, age alone does not seem associated with a patient's tolerance to radiation therapy. Pignon and colleagues[21] looked at 1589 patients, 408 over age 65, in a grouped analysis of the European Organisation for Research and Treatment of Cancer trials and found no difference in overall survival, objective mucosal reactions, long-term toxicity, or weight loss between the groups. There was a significant increase in acute grade 3 to grade 4 toxicity in the elderly group and symptoms related to mucositis.[21] Similarly, Lusinchi and colleagues[22] in a single-institution study, including 331 patients 70 years or older treated with surgery and radiation or radiation alone, found that overall survival was equal in elderly and younger patients. There was severe mucositis rate of 17%. These results of age not having an impact on oncologic outcome or treatment breaks has been seen in multiple other single-institutional retrospective series.[23–25] Alternatively, Allal and colleagues[26] found that although the completion rate was similar between age groups, there were more unplanned breaks in the over-80 group compared with younger patients due to acute toxicity and noncompliance.

Treatment intensification through hyperfractionation has been shown to improve outcomes in head and neck cancer patients.[27] In elderly patients, who are already more sensitive to acute toxicity, this has not been shown effective. Bourhis and colleagues[27] in a meta-analysis, including 6515 patients from 15 trials, found that although this benefit was seen in younger patients, it was not observed in older patients (over age 70 years) and patients with poor performance status. It is believed related to the higher non–cancer-related deaths in this subgroup. Functional acute toxicity is an important concern in this group of patients and comorbid conditions, and functional status should be considered when developing a treatment plan. In addition, supportive measures addressing nutrition, pain, and mucositis are absolutely critical. Finally, as radiation therapy continues to evolve with larger doses to smaller target volumes using techniques, such as intensity-modulated radiation therapy, image-guided radiation therapy, stereotactic body radiation therapy/stereotactic ablative radiotherapy, and proton therapy, tolerance to therapy is anticipated to continue to improve.

CHEMOTHERAPY

The National Comprehensive Cancer Network (NCCN) recommends the addition of chemotherapy to radiotherapy when used as definitive nonsurgical therapy for advanced stage tumors or postoperatively when there is histologic evidence of positive margins or extracapsular extension. There is some evidence, however, that the anticipated survival benefit of chemotherapy may not be seen in older patients. Pignon and colleagues[8] performed a meta-analysis of 93 head and neck cancer clinical trials and found that patients age 71 or older did not benefit from the same 4.5% 5-year survival benefit seen in younger patients when chemotherapy was added to radiation therapy in advanced-stage disease. The investigators believed this was likely related to increased chemotherapy toxicity and non–cancer-related deaths in this subgroup.[8] They also found that age was an independent risk factor for severe late toxicity due to chemotherapy.[8] Argiris and colleagues[28] prospectively evaluated chemotherapy toxicity, response rate, and survival in patients over age 70 compared with younger patients all being treated for recurrent or metastatic head and neck cancer. There was no significant difference in survival or objective response rate between age groups; however, the older patients were significantly more likely to develop severe nephrotoxicity, diarrhea, or thrombocytopenia. A retrospective study of 317 patients with head and neck cancer showed a similar response rate between patients less than age 65 and greater than age 65; however, the older patients had lower overall survival and a high incidence of infections.[29] Despite the lack of prospective data, the retrospective literature is consistent in describing that despite equal rates of response to chemotherapy; the survival benefit may be limited due to the increased toxicity experience by these patients. One retrospective analysis of the National Cancer Database, however, found improved survival with concurrent chemoradiation in patients 71 to 81 years of age with low comorbidity scores and locally advanced disease.[30] The recent introduction of targeted agents, such as cetuximab, has demonstrated improved survival when given with radiation alone and when added to cytotoxic palliative chemotherapy.[31] The decreased toxicity profile of this and other targeted agents has the potential to allow for a greater role for chemotherapy in the management of elderly patients with head and neck cancer.

Regardless, comorbid conditions and increased frailty in older patients require that chemotherapy agents be given with discretion, dose reduction, and close monitoring in select patients. There are dose toxicity calculators available through the Cancer and Aging Research Group.[32] Patients should be closely observed for mucositis and hospitalized for nutritional support if necessary. In addition, clinicians should observe for bone marrow suppression, neurotoxicity, falls, cardiac toxicity, renal toxicity, and insomnia.

ELDERLY SCREENING

Selection of the appropriate therapy for head and neck cancer in an elderly patient requires a thorough understanding of their comorbidities, functional status, values, and social support network. The clinician and patient must decide whether the oncologic benefit relative to life expectancy is outweighed by the toxicity of treatment. There are numerous metrics that have been proposed to standardize this process.

The comprehensive geriatric assessment (CGA) is an in-depth evaluation to assess the overall health, functional status, comorbidities, polypharmacy, nutritional status, cognitive function, psychological status, socioeconomic issues, and elderly syndromes. The CGA can both guide decision making and allow targeted interventions during therapy to minimize adverse outcomes. CGA has been shown the most effective means to risk stratify prior to chemotherapy and predict toxicity.[33] In addition, it has been shown in both prospective and retrospective trials that higher mortality rate is correlated with the identification of multiple CGA deficits.[34,35] Performing a CGA is time consuming and, therefore, not often performed by primary oncologists. In response, screening tools have been developed with the aim of identifying high-risk patients who should undergo CGA, preferably under the care of a geriatrician who is more familiar with the evaluation and interventions available. Some of the proposed screening tools are the abbreviated CGA, Barber Questionnaire, Fried Frailty Criteria, Geriatric 8 (G-8), Groningen Frailty Indicator, Triage Risk Screening Tool, Vulnerable Elders Survey, and Lachs screening test. The results of these tests can be used as an indication for referral for CGA and elderly consultation or used as an independent predictive tool.

Comorbidity is the existence of multiple medical conditions in a patient. Comorbid conditions worsen in severity and number as patients age, and these have been directly shown to decrease survival in cancer patients undergoing appropriate therapy.[36,37] Comorbidities include cardiovascular problems, diabetes, renal insufficiency, dementia, depression, anemia, chronic infections, osteoporosis, pressure ulcers, and prior cancer diagnosis. There are numerous indexes used to quantify comorbidity including the Charlson Comorbidity Index, Cumulative Illness Rating Scale, Older Americans Resources and Services, and Multidimensional Functional Assessment Questionnaire. The ACE-27 is another comorbidity index and has been used in head and neck cancer patients and shown to correlate with overall survival in 310 patients assessed retrospectively.[38]

Functional status is the ability to function independently in society. Decreased functional status has been associated with a higher risk of postoperative complications, a higher risk of need for gastrostomy tube, increased toxicity of chemotherapy, and worse survival.[5,39] Activities of daily living measure the ability to perform basic self-care skills needed to live independently. Instrumental activities of daily living measure the ability to perform complex tasks, such as paying bills, necessary to function independently in society. Both have been correlated with increased post operative complications. Instrumental activities of daily living has been correlated with a higher gastrostomy tube rate[5,39]

Nutritional deficiency is critical to assess in elderly head and neck patients. Head and neck cancer and treatment both can have profound deleterious effects on the ability to masticate and swallow. Elderly patients are already more sensitive to nutritional loss and take longer to restore baseline intake. High-risk patients are identified based on a body mass indix less than 22 or more than 5% weight loss in the previous 6 months.[40] These patients should be started on nutritional supplementation immediately and referred nutritional consultation. In addition, patients undergoing treatment should be monitored for the development of poor nutrition.

The NCCN provides a framework to guide decision making in their online resource: "Older Adult Oncology."[40] In summary, they recommend clinicians initially assess patient age and longevity relative to prognosis of the cancer. If it is deemed necessary to treat, a clinician should ensure the patient goals for treatment are in line with the proposed plan. Finally, a comprehensive elderly assessment or screening tool, such as the G-8, should be performed to stratify risk of toxicity during therapy. If high-risk, palliative or single-modality therapy can be discussed based on patient goals. Otherwise, refer to the NCCN adult guidelines for treatment recommendations.

SUMMARY

Treatment of head and neck cancer in the elderly patient warrants special consideration of patient wishes, anticipated life span, acceptable morbidity, comorbidities, functional status, social support, and nutrition. There has not been shown to be a difference in efficacy of treatment for head and neck cancer in elderly patients. Elderly patients, however, typically have more comorbidities, and are more likely to experience toxicity related to treatment, particularly secondary to chemotherapy. Screening of patient comorbidity and functional status can be achieved with several screening tools that assist in risk stratifying older patients, which can inform a treatment plan that balances treatment toxicity and patient goals.

REFERENCES

1. McGuirt WF, Davis SP 3rd. Demographic portrayal and outcome analysis of head and neck cancer surgery in the elderly. Arch Otolaryngol Head Neck Surg 1995; 121(2):150–4.
2. Audisio RA, Pope D, Ramesh HS, et al. Shall we operate? Preoperative assessment in elderly cancer patients (PACE) can help. A SIOG surgical task force prospective study. Crit Rev Oncol Hematol 2008;65(2):156–63.
3. Szturz P, Vermorken JB. Treatment of elderly patients with squamous cell carcinoma of the head and neck. Front Oncol 2016;6:199.
4. Khafif A, Posen J, Yagil Y, et al. Quality of life in patients older than 75 years following major head and neck surgery. Head Neck 2007;29(10):932–9.
5. Moye VA, Chandramouleeswaran S, Zhao N, et al. Elderly patients with squamous cell carcinoma of the head and neck and the benefit of multimodality therapy. Oncologist 2015;20(2):159–65.
6. Bhattacharyya N. A matched survival analysis for squamous cell carcinoma of the head and neck in the elderly. Laryngoscope 2003;113(2):368–72.
7. Muir CS, Fraumeni JF Jr, Doll R. The interpretation of time trends. Cancer Surv 1994;19-20:5–21.

8. Pignon JP, le Maitre A, Maillard E, et al, MACH-NC Collaborative Group. Meta-analysis of chemotherapy in head and neck cancer (MACH-NC): an update on 93 randomised trials and 17,346 patients. Radiother Oncol 2009;92(1):4–14.

9. Zabrodsky M, Calabrese L, Tosoni A, et al. Major surgery in elderly head and neck cancer patients: immediate and long-term surgical results and complication rates. Surg Oncol 2004;13(4):249–55.

10. Vermorken JB, Specenier P. Optimal treatment for recurrent/metastatic head and neck cancer. Ann Oncol 2010;21(Suppl 7):vii252–61.

11. Warnakulasuriya S. Global epidemiology of oral and oropharyngeal cancer. Oral Oncol 2009;45(4–5):309–16.

12. Milet PR, Mallet Y, El Bedoui S, et al. Head and neck cancer surgery in the elderly–does age influence the postoperative course? Oral Oncol 2010;46(2): 92–5.

13. Kowalski LP, Alcantara PS, Magrin J, et al. A case-control study on complications and survival in elderly patients undergoing major head and neck surgery. Am J Surg 1994;168(5):485–90.

14. Shaari CM, Buchbinder D, Costantino PD, et al. Complications of microvascular head and neck surgery in the elderly. Arch Otolaryngol Head Neck Surg 1998; 124(4):407–11.

15. Clayman GL, Eicher SA, Sicard MW, et al. Surgical outcomes in head and neck cancer patients 80 years of age and older. Head Neck 1998;20(3):216–23.

16. Chaudhary H, Stewart CM, Webster K, et al. Readmission following primary surgery for larynx and oropharynx cancer in the elderly. Laryngoscope 2017;127(3): 631–41.

17. Morgan RF, Hirata RM, Jaques DA, et al. Head and neck surgery in the aged. Am J Surg 1982;144(4):449–51.

18. Bridger AG, O'Brien CJ, Lee KK. Advanced patient age should not preclude the use of free-flap reconstruction for head and neck cancer. Am J Surg 1994;168(5): 425–8.

19. Blackwell KE, Azizzadeh B, Ayala C, et al. Octogenarian free flap reconstruction: complications and cost of therapy. Otolaryngol Head Neck Surg 2002;126(3): 301–6.

20. Dhiwakar M, Khan NA, McClymont LG. Surgery for head and neck skin tumors in the elderly. Head Neck 2007;29(9):851–6.

21. Pignon T, Horiot JC, Van den Bogaert W, et al. No age limit for radical radiotherapy in head and neck tumours. Eur J Cancer 1996;32A(12):2075–81.

22. Lusinchi A, Bourhis J, Wibault P, et al. Radiation therapy for head and neck cancers in the elderly. Int J Radiat Oncol Biol Phys 1990;18(4):819–23.

23. Mitsuhashi N, Hayakawa K, Yamakawa M, et al. Cancer in patients aged 90 years or older: radiation therapy. Radiology 1999;211(3):829–33.

24. Schofield CP, Sykes AJ, Slevin NJ, et al. Radiotherapy for head and neck cancer in elderly patients. Radiother Oncol 2003;69(1):37–42.

25. Zachariah B, Balducci L, Venkattaramanabalaji GV, et al. Radiotherapy for cancer patients aged 80 and older: a study of effectiveness and side effects. Int J Radiat Oncol Biol Phys 1997;39(5):1125–9.

26. Allal AS, Maire D, Becker M, et al. Feasibility and early results of accelerated radiotherapy for head and neck carcinoma in the elderly. Cancer 2000;88(3): 648–52.

27. Bourhis J, Overgaard J, Audry H, et al. Hyperfractionated or accelerated radiotherapy in head and neck cancer: a meta-analysis. Lancet 2006;368(9538): 843–54.

28. Argiris A, Li Y, Murphy BA, et al. Outcome of elderly patients with recurrent or metastatic head and neck cancer treated with cisplatin-based chemotherapy. J Clin Oncol 2004;22(2):262–8.

29. Merlano MC, Monteverde M, Colantonio I, et al. Impact of age on acute toxicity induced by bio- or chemo-radiotherapy in patients with head and neck cancer. Oral Oncol 2012;48(10):1051–7.

30. Amini A, Jones BL, McDermott JD, et al. Survival outcomes with concurrent chemoradiation for elderly patients with locally advanced head and neck cancer according to the National Cancer Data Base. Cancer 2016;122(10):1533–43.

31. Bonner JA, Harari PM, Giralt J, et al. Radiotherapy plus cetuximab for locoregionally advanced head and neck cancer: 5-year survival data from a phase 3 randomised trial, and relation between cetuximab-induced rash and survival. Lancet Oncol 2010;11(1):21–8.

32. Hurria A, Mohile S, Gajra A, et al. Validation of a prediction tool for chemotherapy toxicity in older adults with cancer. J Clin Oncol 2016;34(20):2366–71.

33. Extermann M, Boler I, Reich RR, et al. Predicting the risk of chemotherapy toxicity in older patients: the Chemotherapy Risk Assessment Scale for High-Age Patients (CRASH) score. Cancer 2012;118(13):3377–86.

34. Clough-Gorr KM, Thwin SS, Stuck AE, et al. Examining five- and ten-year survival in older women with breast cancer using cancer-specific geriatric assessment. Eur J Cancer 2012;48(6):805–12.

35. Soubeyran P, Fonck M, Blanc-Bisson C, et al. Predictors of early death risk in older patients treated with first-line chemotherapy for cancer. J Clin Oncol 2012;30(15):1829–34.

36. Meyerhardt JA, Catalano PJ, Haller DG, et al. Impact of diabetes mellitus on outcomes in patients with colon cancer. J Clin Oncol 2003;21(3):433–40.

37. Nanda A, Chen MH, Braccioforte MH, et al. Hormonal therapy use for prostate cancer and mortality in men with coronary artery disease-induced congestive heart failure or myocardial infarction. JAMA 2009;302(8):866–73.

38. Sanabria A, Carvalho AL, Vartanian JG, et al. Comorbidity is a prognostic factor in elderly patients with head and neck cancer. Ann Surg Oncol 2007;14(4):1449–57.

39. VanderWalde NA, Deal AM, Comitz E, et al. Geriatric assessment as a predictor of tolerance, quality of life, and outcomes in older patients with head and neck cancers and lung cancers receiving radiation therapy. Int J Radiat Oncol Biol Phys 2017;98(4):850–7.

40. Older Adult Oncology. 2017. Available at: https://www.nccn.org/professionals/physician_gls/pdf/senior.pdf. Accessed November 20, 2017.

Endocrine Surgery in the Geriatric Population

John Benjamin McIntire, MD[a],*, Susan McCammon, MD[a], Eric R. Mong, BS[b]

KEYWORDS

- Endocrine surgery • Geriatric • Thyroid • Risk stratification

KEY POINTS

- The boom in the elderly population of the United States will undoubtedly impact endocrine surgery.
- Because of the increased likelihood of comorbidities with age, surgical management of these patients can be complex.
- Therefore, careful consideration of surgical indications and risk stratification as well as meticulous perioperative management are paramount.

INTRODUCTION

The elderly constitutes a large, and rapidly growing, portion of the US population.[1] Those who survive to 70 years of age can expect to live an additional 14 years, and those who survive to 80 years of age can expect to live an additional 8 years.[2] The boom in this population subset will undoubtedly impact endocrine surgery. This impact is evidenced by the increased incidence of malignancy and nodular thyroid disease with age; this is particularly concerning, as current thyroid cancer guidelines offer no surgical recommendations that are specific to the geriatric population.[3] Because of increased likelihood of comorbidities with age, surgical management of these patients can be complex. Therefore, careful consideration of surgical indications and risk stratification as well as meticulous perioperative management are paramount.

THYROID DISEASE

In general, data regarding thyroid surgery in the geriatric population are sparse and conflicting, as evidenced by a PubMed review of *geriatric thyroidectomy*, which demonstrated only 23 articles. Although age parameters differ somewhat between

Disclosure: The authors have nothing to disclose.
[a] Department of Otolaryngology, University of Texas Medical Branch, 301 University Boulevard, Galveston, TX 77555-0521, USA; [b] University of Texas Medical Branch, 301 University Boulevard, Galveston, TX 77555-0521, USA
* Corresponding author.
E-mail address: jbmcinti@utmb.edu

studies, the accepted norm is that patients 16 to 64 years old are classified as young, those 65 to 79 years old are classified as elderly, and those 80+ years old are classified as superelderly.[4] There are several single-institution studies that report similar complication rates of thyroidectomy among young and elderly patients. This finding is demonstrated in the data by Passler and colleagues,[5] who concluded that thyroid surgery in patients greater than 75 years old can be performed with low morbidity. In their single-institution study, Tartaglia and colleagues[6] found no significant differences in the incidence of postoperative complications or perioperative mortality when comparing patients greater than 65 years old with a younger cohort. Raffaelli and colleagues[1] specifically studied patients older than 70 years who underwent thyroid surgery and found complication rates similar to historical values. Furthermore, this study cites relatively high rates of thyroid carcinoma and toxic goiter as rationale for an aggressive approach in the geriatric population. Rios and colleagues[7] studied patients older than 65 years who underwent thyroidectomy for goiter and concluded that surgical morbidity and mortality are similar as that of a younger age cohort. Overall these studies suggest that individual risk/benefit analysis, careful preoperative preparation, and close monitoring of comorbidities can mitigate potential increased risk due to age.

Other single-institution studies and seemingly a preponderance of the population-based studies suggest that age may confer an increased risk for thyroid surgery. Seybt and colleagues[8] prospectively analyzed patients undergoing thyroid surgery. Their experimental group was composed of patients older than 65 years, and their control group was aged 21 to 35 years. Like other single-institution studies, they noted a similar rate of complications between the two groups. However, they also noted a trend toward a higher rate of readmission in the elderly group. Unplanned readmission was later studied specifically by Tuggle and colleagues,[3] who used the Surveillance, Epidemiology, and End Results database to identify patients greater than 65 years of age who underwent thyroidectomy. They found that 8% of these patients underwent a 30-day unplanned rehospitalization and that unplanned rehospitalization was associated with increased comorbidity, complication during index stay, and small hospital size. The mean cost of rehospitalization was greater than $5000, and unplanned rehospitalization was significantly associated with death at 1 year. Specifically, survival for unplanned readmission patients at 1 year after discharge was 82%. Additionally, it was noted that large hospitals and postdischarge visits to outpatient providers were associated with a decreased rate of unplanned readmission.

Other studies have sought to evaluate, on a population level, the cost and complications of thyroid surgery in the aging population. Grogan and colleagues,[4] in their prospective cohort study using the National Surgical Quality Improvement Program database, identified an experimental group of nearly 8000 patients who underwent thyroidectomy and a control group of nearly 4000 patients who underwent parathyroidectomy. They stratified the patients by age and evaluated the incidence of nonendocrine complications, such as urinary tract infection, wound infections, cardiac complications, and so forth. With comorbidities controlled, they found that age was an independent risk factor for pulmonary, cardiac, and infectious complications after thyroidectomy. Furthermore, they demonstrated that the elderly cohort was twice as likely, and the superelderly were 5 times as likely, to have a complication compared with young patients. A similarly designed study by Sosa and colleagues[9] evaluated not only clinical outcomes but also economic outcomes of thyroid surgery in the geriatric population. They discovered that high-volume surgeons, defined as performing greater than 30 thyroidectomies per year, had improved clinical and economic outcomes relative to low-volume surgeons. They also found that these high-volume surgeons only performed 29% of the thyroidectomies in the elderly and 15% of the thyroidectomies in the superelderly. These studies highlight the importance of thyroid-ectomy referrals to large centers with high-volume surgeons.

With knowledge that age is a risk factor for thyroid surgery, that unplanned rehospi-talization is relatively common and costly, and that most geriatric thyroidectomies are being performed in the community where cost and complications are high, the ques-tion must be raised whether we should be treating thyroid disease this aggressively in the geriatric population. Jegerlehner and colleagues[10] studied rates of thyroid disease and thyroid surgery over time in Switzerland. They found that the incidence of papillary carcinoma increased dramatically over time, whereas the incidence of nonpapillary carcinoma remained relatively constant; these data are consistent with similar US sta-tistics.[10,11] They also found that the rate of thyroidectomy increased dramatically over time. Finally, they found that the mortality due to thyroid carcinoma remained relatively constant.[10] These findings suggest that the tumors being discovered and treated are the early stage and indolent forms of papillary carcinoma. Furthermore, this suggests that observation may play a role in the management for some patients with thyroid car-cinoma. Ito and colleagues[12] prospectively studied greater than 1000 patients with papillary thyroid microcarcinoma, and these patients were stratified by age and observed for disease progression. In their cohort of patients greater than 60 years of age, less than 2% progressed to clinical disease. These investigators suggested that older patients with low-risk, papillary microcarcinoma may be the best candidates for observation.

Also important is the surveillance and management of nodular thyroid disease. For nodules that do not meet the criteria for fine-needle aspiration on initial imaging, cur-rent guidelines recommend follow-up with repeat ultrasound in 6 to 24 months depending on sonographic characteristics of the nodule. Additionally, for nodules with a benign diagnosis on fine-needle aspiration, it is recommended that these nod-ules undergo follow-up with repeat ultrasound in 12 to 24 months depending on nodule characteristics.[13] If nodules demonstrate stability on a serial ultrasound exam-ination, the value of subsequent imaging is thought to be quite low.[13] Because of a lack of studies that observe nodule growth beyond 5 years, there is no specific recom-mendation for long-term surveillance. In a prospective study of the surveillance of benign thyroid nodules, Durante and colleagues[14] noted that the growth of solitary nodules was inversely associated with age. This finding would give credence to the idea that long-term surveillance of benign thyroid nodules may not be warranted in older individuals.

Knowing that we are not necessarily improving mortality with thyroidectomy and that we can probably observe low-risk disease in some geriatric patients, we must further hone our eyes to those patients who can undergo thyroidectomy safely. The most obvious way of doing this is by looking at their comorbidities. This method be-comes facile with use of modern tools for surgical risk calculation, such as the Amer-ican College of Surgeons' online risk calculator. A less obvious method for predicting surgical complications in geriatric patients is by considering the idea of frailty. Frailty is broadly defined as a state of increased vulnerability resulting from age-associated de-clines in reserve and function across multiple physiologic systems, such that the ability to cope with every day or acute stressors is compromised.[15]

Surgical risk becomes especially important in geriatric patients with increasing pos-sibility or probability of postoperative discharge to somewhere other than home, such as a nursing home or skilled nursing facility. In these cases, it may be helpful to use a tool designed to facilitate shared decision-making, such as the Best Case/Worst Case tool.[16] This tool is a pictographic representation of treatment options that is drawn by the surgeon; it clearly demonstrates the best, worst, and most likely outcome of each treatment option. It has been praised by both surgeons and geriatric patients for its unambiguous representation of treatment options. Decision-making becomes more complex in cases whereby patients lack decision-making capacity, and this is not an unfamiliar scenario when treating geriatric patients. In these cases, a surrogate decision maker is needed. Whether decisions are being made by the patients or their surrogates, many tenets of shared decision-making remain unchanged. Specifically, clinicians should strive to be effective coaches in the decision-making process, rather than authoritative figures.[17] Furthermore, patients, their families, and their surrogates should be encouraged to express what is important to them; they should be informed regarding all reasonable treatment options and the potential consequences of their decisions. In this way, caregivers can be involved in the decision when potentially burdensome care will be their responsibility.

Certain nonsurgical aspects of thyroid disease also come to light in elderly patients. One important consideration revolves around whether thyroid hormone supplementation is needed at the end of life. Hypothyroidism is prevalent in geriatric patients and can lead to impaired cognition and mood. In some cases, this is manifested by confusion, disorientation, and psychosis. This circumstance gives reason to provide thyroid hormone supplementation to augment quality of life in these patients, although specific data on this subject are lacking.[18] Parle and colleagues[19] studied the treatment of subclinical hypothyroidism on cognitive function in geriatric patients and found that thyroid hormone supplementation conferred no cognitive benefit in patients with subclinical disease. Additionally, thyroid hormone supplementation is not without risk; there is a relatively high risk of overtreatment during thyroid hormone supplementation, particularly in the elderly. Older individuals with thyroid hormone excess may experience unintended sequelae, such as atrial fibrillation, weight loss, reduced lean mass, and possibly reduced bone mineral density.[20] Ultimately, this issue will continue to be managed on a case-by-case basis until more specific data are generated.

PARATHYROID DISEASE

Apart from thyroid disease, parathyroid disease is another hurdle faced by many geriatric patients. Primary hyperparathyroidism reaches a peak incidence between 55 and 70 years of age. Although most patients with this disease are asymptomatic or minimally symptomatic, symptoms progress in approximately 40% of patients.[21] As the life expectancy of older individuals continues to increase, these patients are at high risk of developing complications, most notably osteoporosis and fracture. Surgery is not only an effective treatment that can prevent these complications but, for symptomatic patients, parathyroid surgery has also been shown to result in quick, durable, and long-lasting improvement in quality of life.[22] Unfortunately, geriatric patients face similar barriers to parathyroid surgery, as are discussed with thyroid surgery.

Several studies performed in the 1980s noted relatively high morbidity, lengthy hospital stay, and significant mortality for elderly patients undergoing parathyroidectomy.[23] More recent data have been more encouraging, and this is thought to be due to improvements in anesthetic and surgical technique.[23] One improvement in parathyroid surgery is increasing prevalence of the minimally invasive or limited technique. This technique involves use of preoperative localization imaging studies as well as intraoperative parathyroid hormone assay in effort to target and efficiently remove the dysfunctional gland. This technique differs from the traditional bilateral neck exploration; it can allow for shorter operative time, less aggressive dissection, and less surgical morbidity. Using this technique, Pruhs and colleagues[24] demonstrated improved outcomes in geriatric patients when compared with traditional parathyroid surgery.[24]

Additionally, Irvin and Carneiro[25] concluded that limited parathyroidectomy represents a safe and effective treatment option for geriatric patients with primary hyperparathyroidism.

In conclusion, age must be a factor when considering endocrine surgery. Age itself is a risk factor for complications after thyroidectomy, specifically pulmonary, infectious, and cardiac complications. For this reason, in patients with nodular thyroid disease or thyroid microcarcinoma, length of observation must be measured against age and surgical risk. Outcomes of thyroid surgery in geriatric patients can be improved with several measures, including careful preoperative risk stratification based on comorbidities and frailty. It is imperative to have an earnest discussion with patients, their families, and any surrogate decision maker regarding potential outcomes of treatment versus observation, based on the natural history of thyroid disease. It is also important to note that surgical treatment of primary hyperparathyroidism in the elderly is receiving improved success with minimally invasive techniques. As the incidence of endocrine disease and the proportion of elderly patients in our population continue to increase, this topic will undoubtedly escalate in importance over time.

REFERENCES

1. Raffaelli M, Bellantone R, Princi P, et al. Surgical treatment of thyroid diseases in elderly patients. Am J Surg 2010;200:467–72.
2. Gervasi R, Orlando G, Lerose MA, et al. Thyroid surgery in geriatric patients: a literature review. BMC Surg 2012;12(Suppl 1):S16.
3. Tuggle C, Park LS, Roman S, et al. Rehospitalization among elderly patients with thyroid cancer after thyroidectomy are prevalent and costly. Ann Surg Oncol 2010;17:2816–23.
4. Grogan R, Mitmaker EJ, Hwang J, et al. A population-based prospective cohort study of complications after thyroidectomy in the elderly. J Clin Endocrinol Metab 2012;97(5):1645–53.
5. Passler C, Avanessian R, Kaczirek K, et al. Thyroid surgery in the geriatric patient. Arch Surg 2002;137:1243–8.
6. Tartaglia F, Russo G, Sgueglia M, et al. Total thyroidectomy in geriatric patients: a retrospective study. Int J Surg 2014;12:S33–6.
7. Rios A, Rodríguez JM, Galindo PJ, et al. Surgical treatment for multinodular goitres in geriatric patients. Langenbecks Arch Surg 2005;390:236–42.
8. Seybt M, Khichi S, Terris D. Geriatric thyroidectomy: safety of thyroid surgery in an aging population. Arch Otolaryngol Head Neck Surg 2009;135(10):1041–4.
9. Sosa J, Mehta PJ, Wang TS, et al. A population-based study of outcomes from thyroidectomy in aging Americans: at what cost? J Am Coll Surg 2008;206: 1097–105.
10. Jegerlehner S, Bulliard JL, Aujesky D, et al. Overdiagnosis and overtreatment of thyroid cancer: a population-based temporal trend study. PLoS One 2017;12(6): e0179387.
11. Hahn L, Kunder C, Chen M, et al. Indolent thyroid cancer: knowns and unknowns. Cancers of the Head & Neck 2017;2:1–10.
12. Ito Y, Miyauchi A, Kihara M, et al. Patient age is significantly related to the progression of papillary microcarcinoma of the thyroid under observation. Thyroid 2014;24(1):27–34.
13. Haugen B, Alexander EK, Bible KC, et al. 2015 American Thyroid Association management guidelines for adult patients with thyroid nodules and differentiated thyroid cancer. Thyroid 2016;26(1):1–133.

14. Durante C, Costante G, Lucisano G, et al. The natural history of benign thyroid nodules. JAMA 2015;313(9):926–35.

15. Kim S, Brooks A, Groban L. Preoperative assessment of the older surgical patient: honing in on geriatric syndromes. Clin Interv Aging 2015;10:13–27.

16. Kruser J, Nabozny MJ, Steffens NM, et al. "Best case/worst case": qualitative evaluation of a novel communication tool for difficult in-the-moment surgical decisions. J Am Geriatr Soc 2015;63(9):1805–11.

17. Barry M, Edgman-Levitan S. Shared decision making – the pinnacle of patient-centered care. N Engl J Med 2012;366(9):780–1.

18. Joven M. Should the treatment of hypothyroidism be withdrawn in hospice care? J Pain Symptom Manage 2016;52(3):e3–4.

19. Parle J, Roberts L, Wilson S, et al. A randomized controlled trial of the effect of thyroxine replacement on cognitive function in community-living elderly subjects with subclinical hypothyroidism: the Birmingham elderly thyroid study. J Clin Endocrinol Metab 2010;95(8):3623–32.

20. Ruggeri R, Trimarchi F, Biondi B. L-Thyroxine replacement therapy in the frail elderly: a challenge in clinical practice. Eur J Endocrinol 2017;177:R199–217.

21. Morris L, Zelada J, Wu B, et al. Parathyroid surgery in the elderly. Oncologist 2010;15:1273–84.

22. Adler J, Sippel RS, Schaefer S, et al. Preserving function and quality of life after thyroid and parathyroid surgery. Lancet Oncol 2008;9(11):1069–75.

23. Chen H, Parkerson S, Udelsman R. Parathyroidectomy in the elderly: do the benefits outweigh the risks? World J Surg 1998;22:531–6.

24. Pruhs Z, Starling JR, Mack E, et al. Changing trends for surgery in elderly patients with hyperparathyroidism at a single institution. J Surg Res 2005;127:59–62.

25. Irvin G, Carneiro D. "Limited" parathyroidectomy in geriatric patients. Ann Surg 2001;233(5):612–6.

Voice Changes in the Elderly

Sarah K. Rapoport, MD[a], Jayme Meiner, MS[b], Nazaneen Grant, MD[c],*

KEYWORDS

- Voice • Elderly • Impaired vocal function • Presbyphonia

KEY POINTS

- In the elderly, a decline of the voice can lead to introversion and social withdrawal. To compound communication difficulties, many peers of the elderly suffer from age-related sensorineural hearing loss.
- Numerous quality-of-life studies have demonstrated and confirmed how diminished and impaired vocal function causes a rapid deterioration of quality of life in the elderly.
- Stroboscopy is an ideal diagnostic tool for evaluting the dysphonic elderly patient and visualize subtleties in glottic insufficiency and decreased mucosal wave, which hallmark findings in presbyphonia.
- Voice therapy, as well as surgical interventions centered on improving glottic insufficiency, can help to improve voice quality in patients with presbyphonia.

INTRODUCTION

A cry announces our entry to the world on the day we are born. The voice, a sophisticated synchronization between our respiratory, neurologic, and phonatory organs, goes on to serve as our main expression and serves as an indicator of our physical and emotional health throughout the life span. A decline in the voice in the elderly can lead to introversion and social withdrawal. To compound communication difficulties, many peers of the elderly suffer from age-related sensorineural hearing loss.[1] Numerous quality-of-life studies have demonstrated and confirmed how diminished and impaired vocal function causes a rapid deterioration of quality of life in the elderly. Although few longitudinal studies on vocal aging have been published, researchers are driven to quantify the impact of age-related changes on daily life.[2]

The prevalence of dysphonia in the elderly is reported to range from 12% to 47%.[3] In 1 cross-sectional study using the 2012 United States National Health Interview Survey, about 10% of respondents over the age of 65 reported having a problem with their

Disclosure: The authors have nothing to disclose.
[a] Department of Otolaryngology–Head and Neck Surgery, Medstar Georgetown University Hospital, 3800 Reservoir Road Northwest, Washington, DC 20007, USA; [b] Department of Physical Medicine and Rehabilitation, Medstar Georgetown University Hospital, 3800 Reservoir Road Northwest, Washington, DC 20007, USA; [c] Medstar Georgetown University Hospital, 1 Gorman Building, 3800 Reservoir Road Northwest, Washington, DC 20007, USA
* Corresponding author.
E-mail address: nazaneen.grant@medstar.net

Otolaryngol Clin N Am 51 (2018) 759–768
https://doi.org/10.1016/j.otc.2018.03.012
0030-6665/18/© 2018 Elsevier Inc. All rights reserved.

voice. Of these, 1 in 10 sought medical treatment, and of those, only 22% saw an otolaryngologist.[4] Presenting complaints for age-related voice changes can vary greatly, and can include decreased loudness or projection, vocal fatigue, changes in pitch, altered pitch range, and a rough or breathy voice.[5,6] These traits have inevitable overlap with the presentation of many vocal pathologies, so symptoms of aging versus pathologic changes must be distinguished. Various systemic conditions that increase with age may impact the various phonatory organs, including the respiratory system, neurologic control of speech and laryngeal movement, and, of course, the larynx. In this article, we focus on the larynx itself, and explore the normal and gradual impact of organic aging on the voice as well as the pathophysiology of common pathologies that impact voice quality in the elderly.

PATHOPHYSIOLOGIC CHANGES OF AGING VOCAL FOLDS

Clinical studies analyzing the composition of vocal folds were inspired by consistent laryngeal physical examination findings that were described in elderly patients complaining of diminishing vocal performance. In addition to vocal fold bowing and glottic insufficiency, the vocal folds themselves seem to become thin, as though they were deteriorating. As they aged, the vocal folds were losing their elastic and collagenous properties, a process that seemed akin to the changes observed in aging skin. Such alterations in the makeup of the vocal folds contributed to a progressive stiffening and thinning of the vocal folds over time, which was then clinically correlated with loss of vocal efficiency in the aging voice.[7]

The most important part of the vibrating vocal fold is its cover, which consists of a stratified epithelial layer with a superficial lamina propria directly beneath it. The lamina propria is composed of 3 layers, each defined by its histologic makeup. The superficial layer is characterized by a generalized absence of collagen and elastin, the intermediate layer has high levels of elastin with some collagen, and the deep layer is defined by an abundance of threadlike collagen and fiber with low levels of elastin. Together with the extracellular matrix found within the lamina propria, the elastin and collagen within the lamina propria contribute to the viscoelasticity of the vocal folds.[8] Given the robust demand of repetitive, high-frequency impact that the vocal folds incur from phonation, one can imagine how critical collagen's role is to preserve the integrity of the vocal folds through recoil and stretch.[9] The ability of the vocal folds to withstand such repetitive use is critical to their ability to function over the course of years and even decades. To that end, any variation in the amount of elastin and collagen in the lamina propria changes the histology of the vocal fold, which manifests as dysphonia and underscores the pathophysiologic changes of an aging voice.

In 1997, Kiminori Sato and Minoru Hirano pioneered clinical investigations to determine whether changes in the lamina propria of vocal folds could explain physicians' clinical findings of dysphonia. Using light microscopy to examine the elastin fibers in the vocal folds of aging men they observed that the elastin fibers in male vocal folds had degenerated, and as a result the vocal folds seemed to be irregularly fragmented and atrophic. When Sato and Hirano compared these findings to age-matched female vocal folds examined by light microscopy, they found the elastin fibers did not decrease in density. The degeneration of elastin fibers they had observed in the intermediate layer of the lamina propria was specific to male vocal folds.[10] After this discovery of gender-specific changes in vocal fold histology, clinicians began to distinguish between the dysphonia presenting in elderly men from the vocal changes presenting in elderly female patients. As a result, the decrease in elastin in the lamina propria of male vocal folds elucidated the pathologic vocal fold atrophy habitually detected in elderly men presenting with dysphonia.

Detecting how the amount of collagen in vocal folds varied with both the age and gender of a larynx illuminated the underlying mechanism of muscular atrophy noted aging male vocal folds compared with clinically aging female vocal folds, and transformed our understanding of how vocal folds change with gender as well as with age.

As men age, the extracellular matrixes in the vocal folds become more dense, which decreases their pliability. This increase in the density of their lamina propria, caused by an increase in collagen and concurrent loss of elastin, explained the stiffening of the vocal fold noted on stroboscopy in elderly men presenting with dysphonia.[11]

The decades of research delineating the gradual changes of the larynx as it ages serves as the foundation for our understanding of how vocal fold composition varies with both gender and age. An awareness of the biomechanical differences in elderly male and female vocal folds is critical for understanding the vocal traits of an elderly patient.

ASSESSMENT OF THE AGING LARYNX

To ensure a thorough physical evaluation of the patient, the otolaryngologist must rely on a careful laryngeal examination to serve as the cornerstone of his or her clinical assessment. This examination is undertaken in the context of overall health, however, and the status of other aspects of the phonatory apparatus. In first approaching the patient, one may immediately begin a mental assessment of the characteristics of the patient's spoken voice while simultaneously evaluating the patient's physical examination. One can note: Is the patient's voice gravelly or thin sounding? Is there a vocal tremor or other voice breaks? Does it have a wet quality? How is the control of the patient's speech? Does the patient have hemiplegia from a previous stroke? Is the patient walking with a shuffling, Parkinsonian gait? How is their respiratory effort? Might their posture and overall frailty influence the voice? One may even begin imagining which laryngeal examination findings would match the patient's clinical symptoms before conducting a laryngeal examination.

Stroboscopy

Multiple studies reveal that the diagnostic accuracy of a history and physical examination alone, without obtaining a stroboscopy, was as low as 5% in dysphonic patients. When stroboscopy is added, the diagnostic accuracy of an otolaryngologic examination increases to nearly 70%.[12] Observing mobile vocal cords with stroboscopy allows one to detect deficits and changes in the viscoelastic properties of the superficial lamina propria, which would not be possible with laryngoscopy using a steady, non-strobe light source. Given that glottic insufficiency is a hallmark of the mucosal wave in patients with presbyphonia, the use of stroboscopy in elderly patients with voice changes is a critical aspect of their clinical examination.[13] During a stroboscopy examination, a patient holds a microphone against his skin to register the frequency of his own sustained voice. The patient's vocal frequency is programmed to trigger the stroboscopic light source, and ideally the light source then flashes at the frequency of the patient's vocal fold vibrations. Because the vocal vibrations are periodic, a frequency of light will flash at a pace equal to the vocal frequency to produce clear, still images of the vibratory cycle.[14] In voices with increased vocal instability, such as those with increased perturbation or vocal shimmer observed in elderly patients, the pacing of the strobe light has a difficult time syncing with the frequency generated by the vocal folds, resulting in an intermittently blurred image.[15]

This finding itself is diagnostic of a failure of consistent muscular and tissue support to ensure a sustained sound.

Acoustic Analysis

Acoustic analysis by itself does not commonly change clinical management of presbyphonia, but its use is worthy of mention, especially as it can illustrate objectively the tissue changes mentioned earlier in this chapter and can offer additional insight into a patient's underlying pathology. Acoustic analyses of elderly voices have demonstrated that intensity, fundamental frequency, dynamic range, and glitter and shimmer—indexes of glottal perturbation—all shift in the elderly voice when compared with the voice quality of younger controls.[16] Not only do these features change with age, the pattern with which they change varies with gender. For example, the mean fundamental frequency in females ages 20 to 29 is −225 Hz. As women age, the fundamental frequency decreases so that the mean fundamental frequency in women ages 80 to 90 is −195 Hz. In contrast, in men the fundamental frequency of the speaking voice naturally drops until their fifth decade, after which it begins to increase gradually as the men age.[7] Although the medical literature consistently documents that both men and women demonstrate loss of control of pitch and increased variability of fundamental frequency with age, the relationship between age and measures of voice perturbation is less clear. Perturbation measures are relevant clinically to the physician because they can reveal instability of the vocal fold vibration (jitter), irregularity of glottic closure (shimmer), and loss of vocal fold adduction.[17,18]

PRESBYPHONIA

Presbyphonia is the general diagnostic term most commonly given to the dysphonia associated with an aging voice. Given the inherent changes of the vocal folds in elderly patients as well as their persistent symptoms of vocal changes, one might ask whether the vocal fold atrophy with bowing or vocal process prominence observed among elderly patients constitute true laryngeal pathology. Although presbyphonia is the label given to organic changes observed in an aging larynx, whether these changes should be considered pathologic has been debated.[19,20] One study of 57 subjects over the age of 74 sought to distinguish characteristics of elderly patients between those who did and did not endorse a voice complaint. Presbylaryngis was visible on stroboscopy almost equally in the groups, in 87% of dysphonic and 85% of control subjects, but the dysphonic group had more women and had worse aerodynamic measures and overall respiratory strength.

Results of studies evaluating quality-of-life measures in elderly individuals with dysphonia continue to demonstrate a correlation between one's voice quality and overall sense of vitality. Elderly individuals define quality of life broadly, using terms such as physical operation, vitality, general health, mental health, corporal pain, and physical role in life. No matter the definition used, elderly subjects who are aware of their own increased vocal roughness or voice deterioration self-report a tendency to avoid social situations.[7,21] For this reason, encouraging activities such as recreational choir singing, or even prescribing regular speech therapy in an elderly patient at risk of vocal impairments, may be recommendations otolaryngologists should make more regularly to their elderly patients.

Presbyphonia has been likened to sarcopenia, the degenerative loss of skeletal muscle mass quality and strength associated with aging, but the reality is more complex. In fact, presbyphonia can present in elderly patients whose external muscle mass and physical endurance are quite strong.[22] Elderly patients diagnosed with presbyphonia describe their voice changes as hoarseness with or without a breathy quality, reduced vocal projection, an inability to speak as loudly as they once could, decreased maximum phonation time, lower vocal pitch, and occasionally even a vocal tremor.[7,23] These symptoms correlate with the histologic properties attributed to aging vocal folds including a decrease in density and presence of increasing edema within the superficial lamina propria. More specifically, in female patients, we can intuit histologically that the cover of the superficial lamina propria is thickening. Conversely, in male patients we can deduce that the membranous vocal fold is atrophying and shortening owing to a decrease in the elastin density of the vocal fold, and the intermediate lamina propria in thinning resulting in deterioration of contour of the vocal fold.

VOICE THERAPY

Rehabilitation interventions that have proven most effective in these patients include a multidimensional approach combining the subsystems required for functional phonation.[24] Remembering that phonation does not work in isolation, common practices for improving voice efficiency using a multisystem approach include Lee Silverman Voice Training (LSVT), vocal function exercises, and resonant voice training, because these behavioral approaches incorporate respiration, phonation, and resonance into therapy.[25]

The role of speech language pathologists is to combine the patient outcome perspective with evidenced-based therapy. Although voice therapy is not efficacious for all presbyphonia patients, and in for particular patients who have documented phonotrauma, rehabilitation to restore strength to elderly patients with age-related vocal fold bowing and a diagnosis of presbyphonia has been clinically demonstrated and is not to be underestimated. During the natural aging process, there is an element of deconditioning and the vocal folds are not exempt. Historically, there has been limited research conducted on treating the aging larynx; however, there are a few studies that identify behavioral intervention for improving vocal outcomes. In particular, Sauders and colleagues and Gorman and colleagues studied the use of vocal function exercises in patients with presbyphonia. Vocal function exercises were developed by Dr Joseph Stemple and include specific voicing exercises incorporating respiration, phonation and resonance (see **Box 1**). In summary, Dr Stemple's vocal function techniques were found to improve coordination of inhalation and exhalation to support improved vocal flexibility in normal subjects.

Inherent positive reinforcement in patients undergoing speech therapy treatment may be a motivating factor for patients, because therapists have explained that significant changes of phonatory function measures are perceptible relatively early in the treatment sessions and remain stable throughout the course of treatment.[25,26]

Box 1
Vocal functional exercises

1. Sustain /i/ for as long as possible on a comfortable note.

2. Glide from the lowest note to highest note in frequency range using /o/.

3. Glide from the highest note to the lowest note in frequency range using /o/.

4. Sustain C, D, E, F and G above middle C using /o/ for as long as possible.

Exercises should be repeated twice each and completed twice daily.
From Takano S, Kimura M, Nito T, et al. Clinical analysis of presbylarynx–vocal fold atrophy in elderly individuals. Auris Nasus Larynx 2010;374:461–4; with permission.

Quality-of-life standards are shown to have a direct correlation with voice dysfunction in the elderly, and rehabilitative voice therapy is essential for providing improved overall function within activities of daily living. Combining the subsystems of respiration, phonation, and resonance demonstrates effectiveness in improving functional outcomes (**Box 1**).

SURGICAL INTERVENTION

Voice therapy techniques can also be used as an adjunct to surgical intervention, the combination of which possibly is an ideal approach for age-related voice changes,[3] although evidence has yet to prove this as such. Given the glottic insufficiency that characterizes presbyphonia, surgery most often centers on vocal fold augmentation with injectable materials or an implantable prosthesis with a type I thyroplasty.[26]

Injection laryngoplasty specifically has proven to be a minimally invasive, office-based technique ideal for elderly patients who may be too kyphotic to lay supine on an operative table or may have difficulty acquiring medical clearance to undergo general anesthesia for an elective procedure.[27] The procedure medializes atrophic vocal cords or augments nonparalytic glottic incompetence with injectable synthetic materials, such as hyaluronic acid or calcium hydroxylapatite. Likewise, an open medialization procedure using an implant, such as silastic or GoreTex, can improve glottic closure. Augmentation procedures will not improve the tissue quality of the true vocal folds or atrophied musculature, nor will they take into account pulmonary function to increase the power of a patient's voice. However, the opportunity to medialize the vocal folds can result in effective amplification of the patient's voice, thus offering improved voice quality and potentially a restored quality of life for the elderly patient.

EFFECT OF AGING ON THE SINGING VOICE

Singing has been associated with voice stability, greater phonation range, and increased maximal phonation time in elderly patients. These findings spurred researchers to investigate the effect of singing on the aging voice to better comprehend mechanisms that may inhibit vocal decline with age. In an effort to isolate habits that may protect the voice from the natural effects of aging, researchers studied the vocal habits of both professional and recreational singers.[17] If a simple intervention such as singing could potentially prevent or delay the onset vocal decline in the elderly, imagine the valuable impact the latter could have on the quality of life of elderly adults!

For elderly patients who sing recreationally in their church choirs and present to the clinic complaining that they were previously a soprano but are now an alto, one can offer reassurance and advice based on multiple clinical studies. One can bolster a patient's confidence by explaining how data repeatedly shows that elderly singers have significantly higher speaking fundamental frequency than elderly nonsingers during standard reading tasks. So although their singing range may inevitably vary with age, they should not feel discouraged. Rather, one must remind them how continued singing and vocal function exercises can strengthen laryngeal muscles, thus facilitating improved vocal fold vibration.[14]

Although it is unlikely we will ever truly be able to prevent the voice from aging, there is much to gain from studying the habits of patients who defy the normative progression of vocal aging. Although patients with congestive heart disease or pulmonary insufficiency may be limited in their ability to improve their breath control and strengthen their voices through therapeutic rehabilitation, we must use elderly singers who have maintained their vocal bravado as a source of inspiration for motivated elderly patients complaining of breathiness or loss of vocal range.

EFFECT OF PARKINSON'S DISEASE ON THE AGING VOICE

Parkinson's disease (PD) is a debilitating and degenerative motor disorder of the central nervous system. It was estimated that in 2008 that 7 million individuals were diagnosed with PD worldwide. Among those diagnosed, nearly 90% suffered from disease-related communication disorders. In the United States, it is estimated that 2% of the population over the age of 60 is diagnosed with PD, increasing the burden of disease among the elderly.[28] Clinically, PD presents with bradykinesia, rigidity, and a resting tremor.[29] In the largest study examining the laryngeal changes in patients with PD, the effects of PD on the larynx was observed in the early, mid, and late stages of the disease. The factors limiting communication in patients with PD included imprecise articulation, a soft and breathy voice, hoarse quality of voice, monotone voice, and reduced facial expressions secondary to masked facies.[30]

The progressive nature of PD and devastating loss of physical function in patients with the disease is tremendous. Compounding the latter with loss of clear, verbal communication is deemed a particularly handicapping aspect of the disease. We have discussed in this article how dysphonia in the elderly is directly associated with loss of vitality and diminished quality of life. Similar results have been demonstrated for patients with PD. The degradation of laryngeal motor control can have a negative impact on patients with PD and their families long before frank dementia and mental impairment is evident.[31]

In fact, in patients with PD, changes in voice are typically the first notable physical manifestations of disease. Common presentations of speech impairment in Parkinson's patients include loss of prosody, disarticulation, and impaired fluency of sentences. A patient with PD will characterize the changes of his own voice by explaining that his voice sounds softer, breathier, more monotone, and has reduced pitch variation. Stroboscopic laryngeal findings associated with PD include vocal fold thinning and bowing, and the presence of tremors.[30]

Although laryngeal function has been noted to change gradually with the progression of PD, the underlying neural mechanisms of these speech changes are debated. Because inadequate muscle activation is the predominant pathophysiologic explanation for the bradykinesia in patients with PD, it is also thought to be the reason for voice disorders in patients with PD.[32,33] Clinical evidence to support this explanation is seen in patients with PD who are administered levodopa, a pharmaceutical synthetic precursor to dopamine used to reduce the degree of Parkinsonian dystonias by stimulating the production of dopamine in these dopamine-deficient patients. Patients with advanced PD taking levodopa who were tasked with reading repeatedly demonstrated improved vocal comprehensibility, variability in pitch, and loudness, convincing researchers that the tremor and vocal symptoms noted in these patients are associated with the same causes of broader motor dysfunction in patients with PD.[30]

One may also wonder why the voice is often the first notable manifestation of PD. Researchers have posited that the voice changes associated with PD, namely speech intensity and audibility, are largely associated with a more systemic decline in respiratory and laryngeal control. A decreased respiratory driving pressure will reduce the amount of air propelled through the larynx. Concurrent decreased strength and closure of the vocal folds owing to impaired motor function fails to effectively convert the aerodynamic energy of air released by the lungs into acoustic sound.

Although seemingly counterintuitive, patients with PD remain largely unaware of the severity of their voice disorders. Often patients will report feeling as if they are shouting and exerting a great deal of effort to speak at a normal loudness level. LSVT is an intensive form of physical therapy and rehabilitation for patients with PD that trains patients through vocal and respiratory exercises to improve vocal loudness. Patients are directed to undergo four 1-hour sessions for 4 weeks, and those that persevere with the vocal training and vocalization tasks reliably demonstrate improved glottic closure on stroboscopy without simultaneously developing supraglottic hyperfunction.[32,34] The speech therapy and medical literature both recognize that LSVT has diminished success in those patients with more advanced stages of the disease, stressing the need for early recognition of symptoms and implementation of therapy. Additionally, vocal loudness training from LSVT has been anecdotally noted to also improve articulation, facial expression, and swallowing.[32]

In the stages of advances disease where vocal fold bowing or atrophy are noted, procedural intervention with medialization laryngoplasty may serve the patient well by improving and possibly resolving their glottic incompetence. However, in cases of PD, especially in cases of early diagnosis, surgical intervention should be viewed as an adjunct to LSVT and all patients with PD should be treated in a multidisciplinary fashion, including both rehabilitative and interventional methods.

SUMMARY

The impact of aging is as inevitable in the larynx as it is on all other biologic systems. The muscles of larynx have the potential to atrophy, the elastin fibers of lamina propria thin with age, and mucous production diminishes. As a result, the vocal folds fail to approximate appropriately and the stress on once robust vocal folds increases. These changes present as poor voice quality, vocal tension, tremor, and altered fundamental frequency.[24] And even though aging is inevitable, we are gradually amassing data that the negative quality-of-life impact of these voice changes in the elderly can be delayed, inhibited, and improved through vocal function exercises at minimum and procedural intervention such as vocal fold augmentation or medialization thyroplasty when appropriate. Using the patient's symptoms and endoscopic examination as our driving forces for understanding the underlying factors contributing to a patient's chief complaint, we must hold ourselves to the highest standard. Rather than consider presbyphonia as an immutable diagnosis, we must strive to see it as an opportunity to elevate our standard of care and set goals with our patients to work for therapeutic improvement of voice quality whenever possible.

REFERENCES

1. Chiossi JS, Roque FP, Goulart BN, et al. Influence of voice and hearing changes in the quality of life of active elderly individuals. Cien Saude Colet 2014;19(8):3335–42 [in Portuguese].
2. Verdonck-de Leeuw IM, Mahieu HF. Vocal aging and the impact on daily life: a longitudinal study. J Voice 2004;18(2):193–202.
3. Turley R, Cohen S. Impact of voice and swallowing problems in the elderly. Otolaryngol Head Neck Surg 2009;140(1):33–6.
4. Bertelsen C, Zhou S, Hapner E, et al. Geriatric voice problems and treatment in the United States: a national database study. Oral presentation at Fall Voice Conference. Arlington VA, October 13, 2017.

5. Dilley LC, Wieland EA, Gamache JL, et al. Age-related changes to spectral voice characteristics affect judgments of prosodic, segmental, and talker attributes for child and adult speech. J Speech Lang Hear Res 2013;56(1):159–77.

6. Shilenkova VV, Bestolkova OS. Presbiphonia. Age-related changes in the acoustic voice characteristics. Vestn Otorinolaringol 2013;(6):24–7 [in Russian].

7. Sataloff RT, Rosen DC, Hawkshaw M, et al. The aging adult voice. J Voice 1997; 11(2):156–60.

8. Hammond TH, Gray SD, Butler JE. Age- and gender-related collagen distribution in human vocal folds. Ann Otol Rhinol Laryngol 2000;109(10 Pt 1):913–20.

9. Sato K, Hirano M. Age-related changes of elastic fibers in the superficial layer of the lamina propria of vocal folds. Ann Otol Rhinol Laryngol 1997;106(1):44–8.

10. Sato K, Hirano M, Nakashima T. Age-related changes of collagenous fibers in the human vocal fold mucosa. Ann Otol Rhinol Laryngol 2002;111(1):15–20.

11. Hahn MS, Kobler JB, Zeitels SM, et al. Quantitative and comparative studies of the vocal fold extracellular matrix II: collagen. Ann Otol Rhinol Laryngol 2006; 115(3):225–32.

12. Myint C, Moore JE, Hu A, et al. A comparison of initial and subsequent follow-up strobovideolaryngoscopic examinations in singers. J Voice 2016;30(4):472–7.

13. Martins RH, Gonçalvez TM, Pessin AB, et al. Aging voice: presbyphonia. Aging Clin Exp Res 2014;26(1):1–5.

14. Woo P. Stroboscopy. San Diego (CA): Plural Publishing; 2010.

15. Ahmad K, Yan Y, Bless D. Vocal fold vibratory characteristics of healthy geriatric females–analysis of high-speed digital images. J Voice 2012;26(6):751–9.

16. Honjo I, Isshiki N. Laryngoscopic and voice characteristics of aged persons. Arch Otolaryngol 1980;106(3):149–50.

17. Awan SN, Ensslen AJ. A comparison of trained and untrained vocalists on the Dysphonia Severity Index. J Voice 2010;24(6):661–6.

18. Lortie CL, Rivard J, Thibeault M, et al. The moderating effect of frequent singing on voice aging. J Voice 2017;31(1):112.e1-12.

19. Kendall K. Presbyphonia: a review. Curr Opin Otolaryngol Head Neck Surg 2007; 15(3):137–40.

20. Kost K, Parham K. Presbyphonia: what can be done? Ear Nose Throat J 2017; 96(3):108–10.

21. Schneider S, Plank C, Eysholdt U, et al. Voice function and voice-related quality of life in the elderly. Gerontology 2011;57(2):109–14.

22. Oates JM. Treatment of dysphonia in older people: the role of the speech therapist. Curr Opin Otolaryngol Head Neck Surg 2014;22(6):477–86.

23. Gregory ND, Chandran S, Lurie D, et al. Voice disorders in the elderly. J Voice 2012;26(2):254–8.

24. Sauder C, Roy N, Tanner K, et al. Vocal function exercises for presbylaryngis: a multidimensional assessment of treatment outcomes. Ann Otol Rhinol Laryngol 2010;119(7):460–7.

25. Gorman S, Weinrich B, Lee L, et al. Aerodynamic changes as a result of vocal function exercises in elderly men. Laryngoscope 2008;118:1900–3.

26. Takano S, Kimura M, Nito T, et al. Clinical analysis of presbylarynx–vocal fold atrophy in elderly individuals. Auris Nasus Larynx 2010;37(4):461–4.

27. Hamdan AL, Mokarbel R, Dagher W. Medialization laryngoplasty for the treatment of unilateral vocal cord paralysis: a perceptual, acoustic and stroboscopic evaluation. J Med Liban 2004;52(3):136–41.

28. Gibbins N, Awad R, Harris S, et al. The diagnosis, clinical findings and treatment options for Parkinson's disease patients attending a tertiary referral voice clinic. J Laryngol Otol 2017;131(4):357–62.

29. Wu K, Politis M, Piccini P. Parkinson disease and impulse control disorders: a review of clinical features, pathophysiology and management. Postgrad Med J 2009;85(1009):590–6.

30. De Letter M, Santens P, Estercam I, et al. Levodopa-induced modifications of prosody and comprehensibility in advanced Parkinson's disease as perceived by professional listeners. Clin Linguist Phon 2007;21(10):783–91.

31. Warren N, O'Gorman C, Lehn A, et al. Dopamine dysregulation syndrome in Parkinson's disease: a systematic review of published cases. J Neurol Neurosurg Psychiatry 2017;88(12):1060–4.

32. Mahler LA, Ramig LO, Fox C. Evidence-based treatment of voice and speech disorders in Parkinson disease. Curr Opin Otolaryngol Head Neck Surg 2015;23(3): 209–15.

33. Roy N, Kim J, Courey M, et al. Voice disorders in the elderly: a national database study. Laryngoscope 2016;126:421–8.

34. Sackley CM, Smith CH, Rick C, et al. Lee Silverman Voice Treatment versus standard NHS speech and language therapy versus control in Parkinson's disease (PD COMM pilot): study protocol for a randomized controlled trial. Trials 2014; 15:213.

Dysphagia in the Older Patient

Samia Nawaz, MS, Ozlem E. Tulunay-Ugur, MD*

KEYWORDS

- Geriatric • Dysphagia • Older • Presbyphagia • Management • Aging

KEY POINTS

- Dysphagia is an important health concern for elderly populations, intrinsically related to the physiology of aging.
- Dysphagia in the elderly can be misconstrued as a normal part of aging both by physicians and the patients themselves, hence, remaining undetected.
- Dysphagia requires a multidisciplinary approach with involvement of primary care physicians, geriatricians, otolaryngologists, neurologists, gastroenterologists, speech language pathologists, occupational therapists, and nutritionists.

INTRODUCTION

It is estimated that by the year 2050, people aged 65 years or older will account for 25% of the population in developed countries.[1,2] As an overall increase in longevity over the past 50 years is being reported, there is an imminent need to understand changes in physiology with aging and the unique challenges this population faces.[1,3] Dysphagia is an important health concern for elderly populations, intrinsically related to the physiology of aging. A cause of malnutrition, dehydration, aspiration pneumonia, and even asphyxiation, dysphagia affects 7% to 13% of those aged 65 years or older.[1] Particularly vulnerable to dysphagia are individuals afflicted with cognitive dementia or Parkinsonism or those residing in assisted-living facilities; up to 50% of the latter group experiences swallowing difficulties.[1] It is crucial to recognize that dysphagia significantly impacts quality of life, with social and psychological consequences.[4] Often times, dysphagia in the elderly can be misconstrued as a normal part aging both by physicians and the patients themselves, hence remaining undetected. Moreover, the workup of dysphagia can be difficult, as it requires a multidisciplinary approach with involvement of primary care physicians, geriatricians, otolaryngologists, neurologists, gastroenterologists, speech language pathologists, occupational therapists and nutritionists. With dire consequences and mortality, all elderly patients should be assessed for swallowing impairment. This article aims to

Disclosure: The authors have nothing to disclose.
Department of Otolaryngology–Head and Neck Surgery, University of Arkansas for Medical Sciences, 4301 West Markham Street, Slot 543, Little Rock, AR 72205, USA
* Corresponding author.
E-mail address: oetulunayugur@uams.edu

arm the geriatrician and otolaryngologist with the necessary tools in the workup of dysphagia.

Changes in the Physiology of Swallowing with Aging

Dysphagia occurs to some extent in most older adults, usually beginning at 45 years of age.[3] This process, known as presbyphagia, is the result of multiple factors: age-related changes in head and neck anatomy as well as changes in the neural and physiologic mechanisms that control swallowing. Additionally, the prevalence of diseases increase with aging, and dysphagia is a common cofinding of many disease processes or their treatments.

The process of deglutition involves both voluntary and involuntary muscles. Controlled by 6 cranial nerves and about 40 bilaterally innervated muscles, which control the upper digestive tract, swallowing can be divided into 4 distinct phases. These include the oral preparatory, oral transport, pharyngeal, and esophageal phases. Several physiologic changes associated with aging impact these processes, including loss of muscle mass and function, decreased tissue elasticity, cervical spine changes, decreased saliva production, and reduced compensatory capacity of the brain.[2] Holistically, aging slows deglutition and *reduces its efficiency*.

The tongue is the driving force for the initiation of deglutition in normal individuals. The anterior tongue is mostly used for forming a food bolus and, thus, is composed of type II fast-twitch muscle fibers, whereas the posterior tongue is involved in involuntary movements such as propulsion of the food bolus; therefore, it is composed of type I slow-twitch fibers. As we age, *sarcopenia* causes the fibers of lingual musculature to decrease in size and strength.[2] Robbins and colleagues[5] in multiple studies, demonstrated increased lingual isometric pressures and decreased swallow pressures with aging. Additionally, they discovered that swallow pressure reserve and maximum lingual pressures decrease in older adults as compared with those younger than 60 years. They proposed *sarcopenia* as the reason for the impairment of pressure production. Given the role that the tongue plays in swallowing, this is likely one of the important factors that contribute to the increased prevalence of dysphagia in older persons. Tongue strengthening exercises, such as tongue pressing effortful swallow developed by Park and colleagues,[6] have been shown to help healthy older adults increase their maximum tongue pressure, alleviating dysphagia.

Pharyngeal phase changes typically manifest as a delay in initiation of the pharyngeal phase and a delay in laryngeal vestibule closure. These delays put the elderly at a higher risk for aspiration and its consequences. Also contributing to the increased aspiration risk is deterioration of the pharyngoglottal closure reflex. In healthy individuals, this reflex induces adduction of the vocal folds, thereby preventing aspiration if premature spillage of oral content occurs. In individuals with presbyphagia, this reflex is impaired.[7]

In typical elderly individuals, the prevalence of aspiration and penetration remains to be elucidated, as there are conflicting reports, ranging from 0% to 15%.[7] A well-known risk factor is pooling in the pyriform sinuses and resultant overflow into the laryngeal vestibule.

Upper esophageal sphincter (UES) dysfunction can also contribute to postwallow residues. Indeed, esophageal manometry studies on healthy individuals older than 40 years show increased esophageal stiffness and reduced primary and secondary peristaltic pressures.[8] Additionally, Logemann and colleagues[9] demonstrated that younger adults are able to continue the anterior motion of the hyoid bone and move it by 8 mm more once the UES opens, whereas older adults can move the hyoid just enough to open the UES. These differences in hyoid anterior movement indicate the *functional reserve* present in given individuals. Reserve is necessary to assist in recovery when muscle strength is lost.

Contributing Factors

Xerostomia is a common finding in older adults. Although functional salivary production does not seem to change throughout the age spectrum, the elderly have been shown to be very susceptible to the drying effects of certain medications.[10] These medications include but are not limited to anticholinergics, antihypertensives, antiparkinsonian agents, psychotropics, and diuretics. Certain diseases or treatments, such as diabetes mellitus, scleroderma, and radiation, can also result in xerostomia, which can hinder flow of the food bolus and thereby causes its retention in the upper digestive tract.

Other key causes of dysphagia are neurologic and neuromuscular disorders. Stroke, Alzheimer disease, dementia, and Parkinson disease have all been correlated with dysphagia.

Stroke is a prevalent cause of dysphagia with 30% to 65% of the patients experiencing swallowing problems.[11] Poststroke dysphagia can lead to pneumonia, malnutrition, dehydration, and increased length of hospitalization. About 25% of patients with stroke die of aspiration-related complications, such as pneumonia, within 1 year.[12] Dementia has also been linked with dysphagia. Up to 45% of patients with dementia experience swallowing difficulty; therefore, they are susceptible to malnutrition.[13]

ASSESSMENT
History Taking

Early detection is key in order to prevent complications. A detailed history is crucial in evaluating apatients with suspected dysphagia. This history includes inquiring about the consistency, progression, and timing of the dysphagia. Validated questionnaires, such as the 10-Item Eating Assessment Tool, can aid in screening.[14]

It can be difficult to diagnose elderly patients with dysphagia, as it can often be misconstrued as a normal artifact of aging and older patients and families may dismiss it as expected. One of the initial complaints indicating dysphagia can be a feeling of food getting stuck in the throat. They may point to the neck or chest as the area of the food getting stuck. It has been noted that when patients point to the chest as the site of obstruction, they localize the site of the obstruction, whereas patients pointing to the lower neck may have obstruction in the hypopharynx or the lower esophagus.[15] This differentiation may aid in the decision-making during further workup. Other symptoms of dysphagia include unintentional weight loss, coughing while eating, having to wash down food with liquids, increased time needed to be able to complete meals, and increased mucus in the throat. History taking needs to include a thorough understanding of the number of meals eaten during a day, with a detailed description of consistencies of the food eaten, whether aspiration with liquids or solid food occurs, the amount of water and caffeine intake, and weight changes. Social isolation should be questioned as well as how long it takes to finish a meal, the eating environment, and help with preparing meals. Recent pneumonia should be questioned, and a detailed history should be obtained of any recent hospitalizations.

Zenker diverticulum can present with solid food dysphagia. Patients' symptoms of this condition include undigested food regurgitation, borborygmi, nocturnal or postprandial coughing, and halitosis. These patients are at higher risk of aspiration, malnutrition, and dehydration. Cricopharyngeal muscle (CP) dysfunction, which often coexists with Zenker, can also exist alone and can present with dysphagia (mostly to solid food), aspiration, and weight loss.

Patients with head and neck cancer; those afflicted with neurologic disorders, such as Parkinson disease; and patients who have undergone prior surgeries are all at risk for dysphagia.

Physical Examination

A thorough physical examination should be performed with special attention to neurologic, mental, and respiratory systems. If upper aerodigestive system disorders are suspected, it would be appropriate to obtain an otolaryngology consultation to obtain an endoscopic examination of the larynx and pharynx. Flexible laryngoscopy can reveal important findings, such as pooling in the vallecula, vocal fold immobility, laryngeal or hypopharyngeal masses, or incomplete glottis closure. The authors noted that more than 50% of the patients presenting with dysphagia have a positive finding on laryngoscopy ranging from pooling in the pyriform sinuses to glottic gap to vocal fold paralysis.[16]

DIAGNOSTIC TESTING

A good history will generally determine the appropriate testing and further management. Certain complaints can lead to more targeted testing and evaluation. For example, patients pointing to food getting stuck in the midchest will require a gastroenterology consultation and likely an esophagoscopy. Patients complaining of potential aspiration should be evaluated by an otolaryngologist with a swallow study.

Videofluoroscopic Swallowing Study

The videofluoroscopic swallowing study (VFSS), also known as a modified barium study, is the only study that assesses all 4 phases of swallowing. It demonstrates oral and pharyngeal motility problems, ascertains presence of aspiration or penetration, assesses swallow speed, and evaluates postural changes and their effect on aspiration/penetration. This study remains as the *mainstay* of diagnosis and evaluation in patients with dysphagia and is also useful in determining the type of rehabilitative strategies and therapy. **Fig. 1** shows a VFSS revealing a cricopharyngeal bar, which can be a sign of CP spasm. It should be noted that patients without dysphagia can show a CP bar on a VFSS, and the finding itself is not an indication for surgery.

Flexible Endoscopic Evaluation of Swallowing

The flexible endoscopic evaluation of swallowing method uses a flexible laryngoscope to visualize the laryngopharynx as patients are asked to eat different consistencies of food with food coloring. One of its main advantages is that it can be performed bedside, which is especially useful in hospitalized patients. Additionally, there is no exposure to radiation. However, this method is limited in the assessment of the oral and esophageal phases and is limited in assessing pharyngeal contraction. It is very useful in assessing the presence of penetration, aspiration, residue in the vallecula and pyriform sinuses, and premature spillage onto the laryngeal vestibule.

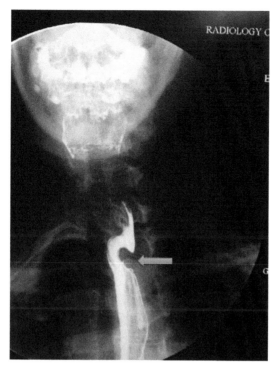

Fig. 1. The arrow points to a cricopharyngeal bar.

Esophagogram

If the cause of dysphagia seems esophageal rather than oropharyngeal in nature, esophageal function should be evaluated. This evaluation can be done through several methods, including an esophagram, which should be considered a first-line measure. This can elucidate pathology, such as webs, strictures, and ulcers. In patients with a suspected Zenker diverticulum or CP spasm, ideally a VFSS with follow-through esophagogram should be obtained.

Pharyngeal and Esophageal Manometry

Upper and lower esophageal sphincter function, pharyngeal strength and contraction duration, completeness of UES relaxation, and the coordination of pharyngeal contractions and UES relaxation can be assessed.

TREATMENT

The main purpose of dysphagia management is the prevention of aspiration and malnutrition as well as its consequences. Once safe swallowing is obtained, the ensuing aim is to improve quality of life. A multidisciplinary approach should be employed, including nurses, dietitians, speech and language pathologists, primary care physicians, neurologists, gastroenterologists, and otolaryngologists. The mainstay of management is rehabilitative and consists of swallowing therapy and diet modifications.[16]

Surgical Management

Cricopharyngeal spasm and Zenker diverticulum (**Figs. 2** and **3**) are mainly diseases of the older patients and are amenable to surgical management. Additionally, there

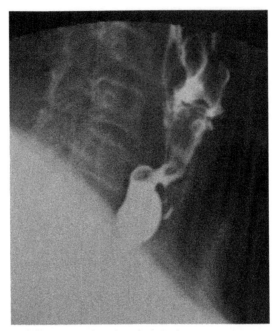

Fig. 2. Videofluoroscopic finding of Zenker diverticulum.

are numerous surgical procedures described for the management of chronic, intractable aspiration, which is beyond the scope of this article. The selection of the surgical candidate in CP spasm and Zenker diverticulum remains elusive, and there are no accepted guidelines for the management of these patients. Each patient is assessed individually, with factors such as weight loss and risk of aspiration pneumonia driving the decision-making. These disorders significantly affect quality of life, as patients need to significantly alter the consistencies of the food they eat, commonly cough all day because of persistent mucus in the hypopharynx, and have poor sleep quality due to continued coughing at night with the secretions

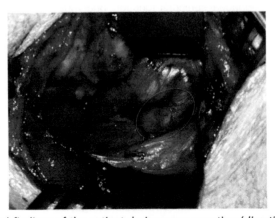

Fig. 3. The surgical findings of the patient during open resection (*diverticulum circled*).

retained in the pyriform sinuses or Zenker pouch, spilling into the laryngeal vestibule. Medical comorbidities of patients are also taken into consideration, as perioperative risk stratification can alter the type of treatment offered. In patients who are not good surgical candidates because of medical comorbidities, less invasive options can be proposed, which include placement of a feeding tube. Furthermore, there is significant proliferation of office-based procedures with minimal sedation or no sedation within otolaryngology. Transnasal esophagoscopy is now used by most otolaryngologists and enables diagnostic esophagoscopy, esophageal dilatation, biopsies, and injections to be performed on nonsedated patients in the clinic. Similarly, botulinum toxin injection for CP spasm can be performed with electromyography guidance in the clinic in patients who are at high risk for complications under general anesthesia.

In a recent systematic review in which the authors evaluated the success and complication rates of UES dilatation, botulinum toxin injection into the CP muscle (**Fig. 4**), and CP myotomy for patients with CP spasm, they demonstrated comparable complication rates but increased success as the invasiveness of the procedure increases. Thus, myotomy was noted to show significantly better outcomes. When open versus endoscopic myotomy was compared, it was noted that endoscopic myotomy had better results with less complications. Hence, patients with suspected CP dysfunction would benefit from an otolaryngology consultation to enable discussion of surgical options. Although patients with idiopathic CP spasm generally respond better to treatment, CP dysfunction due to stroke and head and neck radiation can also benefit from surgical intervention and should be evaluated.[17]

Multiple surgical techniques exist for the management of Zenker diverticulum that can broadly be classified into open versus endoscopic procedures. As discussed earlier, there are no accepted guidelines; the treatment method depends on the surgeon's preferences as well as the anatomy of patients, comorbidities, the size of the diverticulum, and symptoms. Surgical treatment options range from botulinum toxin injections and CP dilatation or myotomy to endoscopic-assisted stapling of the diverticulum (**Fig. 5**), laser-assisted myotomy, and open diverticulectomy.

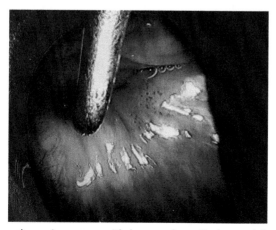

Fig. 4. CP during endoscopic surgery with laryngeal needle inserted for botulinum toxin injection.

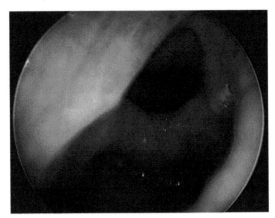

Fig. 5. Endoscopic view of Zenker diverticulum.

Nonsurgical Management

Swallowing therapy is the mainstay of dysphagia management. Swallowing rehabilitation aims to improve physiology through exercises. These exercises aim to minimize or prevent dysphagia-related morbidities and improve impaired swallowing physiology. The most commonly used strategies are postural adjustments, swallowing maneuvers, and dietary modifications. Swallow studies are used to assess the effectiveness of proposed maneuvers and are also used to provide patients with feedback on the effectiveness of the therapy.

Enteral Feeding

Placing a percutaneous endoscopic gastrostomy (PEG) tube is a difficult decision when caring for patients with dysphagia, especially if they lack decision-making capacity. However, use of PEG tubes is expanding; its indications include neurologic and psychiatric disorders, malnutrition, as well as prolonged illness. Patients with head and neck cancer often require PEG to prevent malnutrition.

Approximately 30% of PEG tubes are placed in patients with dementia, whereas 10% of institutionalized elderly patients are PEG tube fed. It is very important to note that PEG placement does not necessarily prevent aspiration pneumonia nor does it reduce the risk of pressure sores or improve survival and function.[18] Other research has confirmed that nutritional markers, such as albumin, do not change with PEG placement.[19] Mortality among tube-fed patients is not insignificant, with patients with dementia having the worst prognosis. Therefore, decisions to place a PEG tube should always be individualized and an interdisciplinary team approach should be used.

SUMMARY

Dysphagia in the older adult is a challenging problem and necessitates a team approach. The key to effective management is recognition. Patients tend to dismiss their symptoms as normal aging; therefore, early diagnosis depends on the diligence of the primary care doctors. No diagnostic technique can replace the benefits of a thorough history, with a detailed understanding of nutritional status and aspiration risk. Although one of the main goals in management is to ensure safe swallowing, the impact of a nonoral diet on the quality of life of patients should not be underestimated; all other treatment options should be exhausted before PEG placement.

REFERENCES

1. Logrippo S, Ricci G, Sestili M, et al. Oral drug therapy in elderly with dysphagia: between a rock and a hard place! Clin Interv Aging 2017;12:241–51.
2. Pitts LL, Stierwalt JAG, Hageman CF, et al. The influence of oropalatal dimensions on the measurement of tongue strength. Dysphagia 2017;32(6):759–66.
3. Namasivayam-MacDonald AM, Morrison JM, Steele CM, et al. How swallow pressures and dysphagia affect malnutrition and mealtime outcomes in long-term care. Dysphagia 2017;32(6):785–96.
4. Nakato R, Manabe N, Kamada T, et al. Age-related differences in clinical characteristics and esophageal motility in patients with dysphagia. Dysphagia 2017;32: 374–82.
5. Robbins J, Humpal NS, Banaszynski K, et al. Age-related differences in pressures generated during isometric presses and swallows by healthy adults. Dysphagia 2016;31:90–6.
6. Park D, Lee HH, Lee ST, et al. Normal contractile algorithm of swallowing related muscles revealed by needle EMG and its comparison to videofluoroscopic swallowing study and high resolution manometry studies: a preliminary study. J Electromyogr Kinesiol 2017;36:81–9.
7. Allen JE, White CJ, Leonard RJ, et al. Prevalence of penetration and aspiration on videofluoroscopy in normal individuals without dysphagia. Otolaryngol Head Neck Surg 2010;142:208–13.
8. Gregersen H, Pedersen J, Drewes AM. Deterioration of muscle function in the human esophagus with age. Dig Dis Sci 2008;53:3065–70.
9. Logemann JA, Pauloski BR, Rademaker AW, et al. Temporal and biomechanical characteristics of oropharyngeal swallow in younger and old men. J Speech Lang Hear Res 2000;43:1264–74.
10. Ney DM, Weiss JM, Kind AJ, et al. Senescent swallowing: impact, strategies, and interventions. Nutr Clin Pract 2009;24:395–413.
11. Mann G, Hankey GJ, Cameron D. Swallowing function after stroke: prognosis and prognostic factors at 6 months. Stroke 1999;30:744–8.
12. Martino R, Foley N, Bhogal S, et al. Dysphagia after stroke: incidence, diagnosis, and pulmonary complications. Stroke 2005;36:2756–63.
13. Horner J, Alberts MJ, Dawson DV, et al. Swallowing in Alzheimer's disease. Alzheimer Dis Assoc Disord 1994;8:177–89.
14. Cheney DM, Siddiqui MT, Litts JK, et al. The ability of the 10-item eating assessment tool (EAT-10) to predict aspiration risk in persons with dysphagia. Ann Otol Rhinol Laryngol 2014;124:351–4.
15. Edwards DA. Discriminative information in the diagnosis of dysphagia. J R Coll Physicians Lond 1975;9:257–63.
16. Kocdor P, Siegel ER, Giese R, et al. Characteristics of dysphagia in older patients evaluated at a tertiary center. Laryngoscope 2015;125:400–5.
17. Kocdor P, Siegel ER, Tulunay-Ugur OE. Cricopharyngeal dysfunction: a systematic review comparing outcomes of dilatation, botulinum toxin injection and myotomy. Laryngoscope 2016;126:135–41.
18. Finucane TE, Christmas C, Travis K. Tube feeding in patients with advanced dementia: a review of evidence. JAMA 1999;282:1365–70.
19. Cervo FA, Bryan L, Farber S. To PEG or not to PEG: a review of evidence for placing feeding tubes in advanced dementia and the decision making process. Geriatrics 2006;61:30–5.

The Effects of Reflux on the Elderly

The Problems with Medications and Interventions

Abie H. Mendelsohn, MD

KEYWORDS

- Laryngopharyngeal reflux • Geriatric • Laryngitis • Proton pump inhibitor
- Treatment

KEY POINTS

- The world's population is aging at an alarming rate, so otolaryngologists need to be aware of the issues related to diagnosis and treatment of this patient group.
- Elderly patients are less likely to experience typical reflux symptoms of heartburn or acidic regurgitation; nonspecific complaints of subjective dysphagia and throat discomfort may be the only presenting symptom.
- Reflux symptoms in the elderly are not reliable to suggest severity of disease; therefore comprehensive evaluation should be considered.
- Proton pump inhibitors are no longer associated with increased risk of dementia, although their effectiveness in controlling symptoms is equivalent to reflux lifestyle and diet modifications alone.
- Care should be taken when recommending laparoscopic antireflux surgery, because elderly patients may be more likely to suffer relapse of their symptoms than younger patients.

INTRODUCTION: REFLUX, LARYNGOPHARYNGEAL REFLUX, AND GASTROESOPHAGEAL REFLUX DISEASE

Throat discomfort is one of the most common presenting symptoms to the otolaryngologist, and many times this symptom is caused by poorly controlled laryngopharyngeal reflux (LPR). LPR can occur in conjunction with classic gastroesophageal reflux disease (GERD) or without.[1] Although LPR has perhaps been used too often to explain chronic throat discomfort, it is undoubtedly a true diagnostic cause from which many patients suffer. The precise burden of this disease is unclear due to the various definitions ascribed to its diagnosis. For instance, diagnosing LPR based on

Disclosure Statement: The author has nothing to disclose.
Department of Head and Neck Surgery, UCLA Voice Center for Medicine and the Arts, 200 Medical Plaza, Suite 550, Los Angeles, CA 90095, USA
E-mail address: Amendelsohn@mednet.ucla.edu

symptom burden would lead to a drastic overestimation of disease incidence.[2] Combining laryngoscopy and symptom-based indices (such as the *Reflux Symptoms Index*[3]) can improve diagnostic accuracy but is far from flawless. Accurate diagnosis requires objective pH monitoring, although there is currently a need for standardization regarding the precise diagnostic thresholds.[4] Nevertheless, by way of proxy to understand the disease burden specifically of LPR, the substantial disease burden of GERD may be investigated. Between 25 and 75 million Americans suffer from GERD, and approximately 13% of US citizens take an anti-GERD medication at least twice a week.[5] Annual per-patient cost for treating GERD is an average of $971,[6] with overall US disease-specific expenditure estimated at $12.1 billion.[7] To make matters worse, patients with extraesophageal symptoms of GERD, such as LPR, have a 5 times higher economic burden with combined costs of consultations, diagnostic procedures, and prescriptions totaling $5438 per patient.[8]

INTRODUCTION: THE AGING POPULATION

Accurately diagnosing LPR is challenging enough but is now complicated by a rapidly aging population. Based on the US Census Bureau 2015 report entitled, "An Aging World," this is a time of substantial transition.[9] America's elderly population of 65 and over will double over the next 30 years. Whereas there are currently 48 million Americans in this age group, there will be more than 88 million by 2050. The number of elderly people is expected to increase by more than 60% in the next 15 years. Worldwide, there will be an *annual* average increase of 27.1 million elderly people. One cause of these astonishing statistics is the improvement in life expectancy, growing from a worldwide level of 68.6 years in 2015 to 76.2 years of age by 2050. Not only will there be an increase in overall number of elderly people, but with the relative diminishing birthrate (as compared with previous generations), there will also be a dramatic increase of the elderly's share in the overall population. Currently 8.5% of the estimated 7.3 billion people in the world are 65 and over. By 2050, this percentage will skyrocket to 16.7% of the estimated 9.4 billion people in the world.[9] The otolaryngologist is now expected to not only correctly manage their patients but also be keenly aware of the issues specific to the aging population.

INTRODUCTION: THE IMPACT OF AGING ON REFLUX

The incidence of reflux most likely increases as one ages. In a collection of more than 3000 elderly patients, almost 22% presented to their primary care office with acid reflux–related symptoms.[10] Moreover, older patients do not experience the typical set of reflux-related symptoms of heartburn or acid regurgitation. Instead, older patients are more likely to present with GERD-related esophagitis with anorexia, weight loss, anemia, vomiting, and dysphagia.[11] This last symptom of chronic subjective dysphagia should be of particular interest to the otolaryngologist because more than one-third of patients older than 75 have some extent of oropharyngeal dysphagia.[12] In fact, the otolaryngologist needs to be vigilant regarding the diagnosis of reflux because it is also common for elderly patients with objective evidence of esophageal erosion to have either nonspecific symptoms or no symptoms at all.[11] Therefore, without a high index level of suspicion, sequelae of undiagnosed reflux may go untreated. Case in point for patients with reflux, the presence of Barrett metaplasia is significantly elevated in patients older than 60 years (25%, compared with 15% of younger patients).[13]

Why should age increase the incidence and severity of reflux disease? Many physiologic mechanisms have been suggested to explain this effect. First, as one ages, there is a breakdown of the natural antireflux barrier. Transient lower esophageal sphincter (LES) relaxation is an event in which the gastric opening to the esophagus is relaxed without a corresponding swallow. Transient LES relaxation is the most common pathophysiologic mechanism of reflux episodes. Although an aging esophagus is unlikely to produce increased transient LES relaxations,[14] elderly patients are much more likely to be taking one or more medications that can promote these inappropriate relaxations. Medications that have been shown to increase the frequency of transient LES relaxation events include nitrates, calcium blockers, benzodiazepines, anticholinergics, antidepressants, and lidocaine. A separate method of a diminished antireflux barrier is a hiatal hernia. The presence of a herniated gastric cavity through the diaphragm hiatus increases reflux independently or together with transient LES relaxations events,[15] and the incidence of hiatal hernias increases with age older than 60.[16] Both mechanisms of barrier breakdown result in elderly patients with poor reflux control.

The other pathophysiologic mechanism explaining the increased incidence of reflux in the elderly is a diminished clearance of esophageal acid. Several effectors cause this poor clearance of refluxate. Esophageal motility provides appropriate muscular contractions to propel food boluses to the stomach and is also critical to return refluxate back to the gastric mucosa. Even without formal diagnoses of esophageal motility disorders such as achalasia, elderly patients are seen to hold significantly longer duration of reflux events despite not necessarily holding more frequent reflux events as compared with younger patients.[17] It is seen that acidic refluxate stays in the esophagus longer in the elderly because of poor esophageal propulsion toward the stomach. In addition, minor salivary glands within the upper gastrointestinal tract produce and secrete bicarbonate capable of neutralizing refluxed acid. Although salivary volume and bicarbonate concentration are unchanged when comparing healthy elderly patients to younger cohorts, elderly patients exhibit a remarkably poorer responsiveness of bicarbonate production, which should be triggered when exposed to esophageal acidic environments.[18] Therefore, with diminished esophageal clearance and inefficient neutralization of the acid, elderly patients are at risk for more severe effects of reflux as was mentioned earlier with the increased incidence of Barrett among the elderly.[13]

REFLUX IN THE ELDERLY: EVALUATION

There is an important change when evaluating reflux symptoms between the younger patient and the elderly patient. Specifically, when encountering a patient with signs and symptoms consistent with either LPR or GERD, many practitioners will favor initiating empiric therapy before recommending an invasive workup. Younger patients who either have a poor response to the therapy or are unable to be weaned off from conservative behavioral and medical therapy are then usually referred for comprehensive gastroesophageal workup. In patients 65 and over, wherein the symptoms are generally less than specific and are not reliable to suggest severity of disease, comprehensive evaluation should be considered upfront before empirical medical management. Although this change in approach toward early invasive evaluations may appear paradoxically risky in the elderly, misdiagnoses and underdiagnoses can represent an equally if not greater risk for these patients.

The gold standard for LPR diagnosis is the presence of inappropriate drops of pH in the pharynx. The classic method of assessing pharyngeal pH levels is the placement of dual pH probes, one just above the LES and one with the lateral oropharynx.[1] An LPR event is commonly defined when pH in the pharyngeal sensor drops greater than 4 during, or immediately after, distal acid probe exposure. LPR is confirmed when total pharyngeal acid exposure time is more than 1%.[19] This evaluation method is accurate in assessing the esophageal pH homeostasis, and it does attempt to correlate the findings with symptoms by having patients document or signal when they experience the reflux sensations.

However, true understanding of the intraesophageal state is best achieved with manometry with multichannel intraluminal impedance combined with pH-monitoring studies.[19] This technique uses changes in resistance to alternating current between a series of metal electrodes and the esophageal mucosa electrolytes. Refluxed gas and liquid, or swallowed boluses, will alter the electrical conductivity of the system and will be evidenced on the graphical display. When combined with pH transducers within the wire, it makes it possible to give a more detailed description of the function of the esophageal physiology. However, despite the physiologic evaluation, a visual inspection of the upper digestive tract is also required to assess for reflux sequelae.

Formal upper gastroesophagoscopy can be combined at the time of sedation for the manometry/impedance placement. Alternatively, many laryngologists prefer in-office transnasal esophagoscopy (TNE) for visualization of the upper digestive tract mucosa. TNE performed under local anesthesia alone can be an excellent immediate and safe option for those patients having already undergone the required diagnostic workup for reflux. TNE, or standard gastroesophagoscopy, should be strongly recommended to reflux patients of all ages because 20% of LPR patients will have evidence of esophageal lesions.[20]

REFLUX IN THE ELDERLY: MEDICAL MANAGEMENT

Once the diagnosis is established, reflux must be treated to minimize symptoms and reduce the sequelae of untreated disease. Integral within any medical therapy strategy is the implementation of behavioral and lifestyle modifications. Changes in lifestyle may be as effective in controlling episodes of heartburn and acid regurgitation in the elderly, as is seen in the young patient. In fact, emphasis on lifestyle modifications may be particularly appropriate in the elderly, in whom polypharmacy may already be a significant issue. Important behavioral changes include weight loss, smoking cessation, and alcohol avoidance. Important dietary changes restrict chocolate, citrus fruits and juices, carbonated beverages, spicy foods, tomato-based products, red wines, caffeine, and late-night meals. Such behavioral changes that appear to be an independently significant variable in determining response to medical therapy in fact may lead to equivalent levels of symptom improvements as gained with prescription medication.[21]

Antacids are medications designed to neutralize gastric acid and are a frequently self-administered medication class for symptom relief. There are many formulations of the classic antacids, including sodium bicarbonate and calcium carbonate. However, not only are these medications poorly effective in treating reflux disease but also they hold significant implications within the elderly population. Sodium bicarbonate tablets will be contraindicated for patients with hypertension or on a salt-restrictive diet. Calcium- and aluminum-based antacids will cause constipation in an elderly population in whom constipation is already a prevalent disorder.[10] Hypercalcemia and interference with drug metabolism are other important considerations with chronic antacid use. Patients who experience symptomatic relief on antacids should be transitioned to more reliable and efficient treatment options. The exception to this rule is alginate preparations, which can be used for long-term antireflux management. Although Gaviscon contains many classic antacid preparations (sodium bicarbonate, calcium carbonate, magnesium carbonate), it is the alginate that particularly sets it apart in this medication class. The alginate will create a foam within the gastric cavity and form a physical barrier limiting refluxate into the esophagus. Its utility has been evaluated in the treatment of LPR with promising results.[22]

Proton pump inhibitors (PPIs) are generally considered the mainstay of reflux medical management. However, in a double-blind randomized placebo study, Steward and colleagues[21] were unable to identify any difference in symptoms or objective pH probe effects between lifestyle modifications with PPIs versus lifestyle modifications with placebo. In another double-blind randomized placebo study, Reichel and colleagues[23] were able to show LPR symptom improvement after 3 months of twice-daily PPI therapy versus placebo. Importantly, Reichel and colleagues used symptoms and laryngoscopy findings alone to define LPR as well as offered no lifestyle modifications to either group, which may severely hamper the clinical applicability of their findings. Moreover, specifically, the otolaryngologist treating voice, or hoarseness, as the primary LPR symptom should also be cautious regarding the effectiveness of PPI therapy. Fass and colleagues[24] designed their double-blind placebo study to compare voice parameters on hoarse LPR patients confirmed with pH probe testing and failed to see any difference between placebo and twice-daily PPIs. Therefore, although PPIs are commonly used in treating reflux disease, appropriate limited expectations should be taken regarding their overall utility, particularly without lifestyle and diet modifications.

Measuring the effectiveness of PPIs is especially of interest in light of the recent suggestion that chronic PPI use can lead to increased risk of dementia, a highlighted concern in the elderly for whom dementia is most prevalent. The connection between dementia and PPI use had been initially suggested by 2 large German studies. In the first study, with a cohort review of elderly patients, investigators saw a significant multivariate association between the presence of dementia and chronic PPI administration.[25] The second, published the following year, looked at a larger patient group through government claims database analysis. Use of PPI was associated with an increased risk of incident dementia.[26] However, in order to establish voracity to this claim, a larger Finnish nested investigation using prospective trial patient data analyzed via a case-control study design concluded that there was no increased risk or association between PPI and the presence of Alzheimer dementia.[27] This lack of connection between PPI and dementia has been corroborated,[28] and even patients on PPIs have been suggested to have a lower risk profile for dementia.[29] In all, current data support the safety of PPI use from dementia.

Histamine 2 blockers, more accurately termed histamine 2 receptor antagonists (H$_2$RAs), are generally thought to be a second-line medical option behind PPIs mainly because of the shorter duration of action requiring twice-a-day dosing. Not forgetting that PPIs have also been shown to be maximally effective on twice-a-day dosing, their duration of action is still longer than H$_2$RAs.[20] Elderly patients on chronic H$_2$RAs use may be at risk for mental status changes (typically described as acute confusion), especially in the presence of some renal or liver impairment.[30] The H$_2$RA cimetidine can interfere with liver enzyme metabolism, which can affect patients on medications, including propranolol, clozapine, cyclobenzaprine, and warfarin. Moreover, the utility of the H$_2$RA ranitidine has shown questionable efficacy in treating reflux as a single agent.[31] As such, the use of H$_2$RAs is generally as a backup second agent with breakthrough or incompletely treated symptoms while on optimal PPI therapy.

Prokinetic agents are a range of medications that increase the motility of the gastrointestinal tract. This group of medications has historically been marred by an increased side-effect profile, which holds specific concern for the elderly population. Cisapride, a serotonin 5-HT$_4$ receptor agonist, had shown initial promise as a reflux therapy option, but ultimately was taken off the market because of lethal side effects, including prolonged QT syndrome.[32] Metoclopramide, a dopamine antagonist, should not be used in the elderly because of side effects in up to one-third of patients, including muscle spasm, agitation, drowsiness, confusion, and tardive dyskinesia. Tegaserod, another 5-HT$_4$ agonist, did show improvement in reflux patients and improved esophageal sphincter relaxation events.[33] However, because of increased association with stroke and heart attacks, the US Food and Drug Administration pulled their approval in 2007. Given their poor safety profile and limited demonstrated benefit in LPR, prokinetics should not be used by the otolaryngologist for elderly reflux patients.

REFLUX IN THE ELDERLY: SURGERY AND NEW INNOVATIONS

Surgery is indicated when medical management is insufficient to control symptoms or objective measures of reflux. Standard of care is laparoscopic antireflux surgery with fundoplication.[34] Criterion for surgical candidacy requires objective testing proving inappropriate acid reflux as well as ensuring normal esophageal motility. The motility studies, generally performed with wire manometry, can rule out esophageal achalasia, which can mimic any of the symptoms of both GERD and LPR. Effectiveness of laparoscopic antireflux surgery has been investigated through multiple randomized control trials. The LOTUS trial compared laparoscopic surgery versus esomeprazole medical management and saw equivalent excellent control of symptoms, although surgical patients had some surgical-related complaints.[35] A 5-year follow-up study on the REFLUX trial, which randomized reflux patients to continued medical PPI management versus laparoscopic surgery, revealed symptom control equal to that of medical therapy and that only 15% of the surgery patients were taking PPI at 5 years.[36] Three-year follow-up on another randomized control trial not only corroborates the long-term symptom control but also suggests that laparoscopic surgery may be more effective in reflux symptom control than medical management.[37]

Overall, it would appear that surgery could be an excellent option for elderly reflux patients, particularly when polypharmacy is present. Nevertheless, emerging data suggest that patients older than 60 have an increased risk of reflux symptom recurrence after laparoscopic surgery. In the recent study of more than 2600 patients undergoing antireflux surgery, 17.7% were failures. Age older than 60 offered a significant and substantial hazard ratio of 1.4 times risk for failure.[38] Although this finding of age as a risk factor for surgical failure has not been consistently identified,[39,40] understanding this relationship will be important given the poor outcomes following revision laparoscopic antireflux surgery.[41] At this time, more data are needed to evaluate outcomes of traditional laparoscopic surgery in the elderly reflux patient. Surgery should be considered only when indications are met for failure of medical management.

LES augmentation procedures have been proposed as a minimally invasive alternative to laparoscopic fundoplication. Although many procedures and devices that had been quite popular several years ago have now either fallen out of favor or are completely unavailable, LINX (Torax Medical, Shoreview, MN, USA) has been showing some promising results. LINX is a series of implantable interlinked magnetic titanium beads. The beads are connected by wires that define the distance the beads can separate. Each bead can move independent of the other beads. The device is made specifically to accommodate individual measurements of the external diameter of the LES. The device is inserted laparoscopically around the outside of the LES.

When a patient swallows a food bolus, the peristaltic pressure overcomes the magnetic attraction and the device opens. As the peristaltic pressure drops, the device is drawn closed by the magnets. In a prospective, multicenter, single-arm, clinical trial, patients aged 18 to 75 saw reliable improvements in quality of life. Eighty percent had complete cessation of the use of PPIs at the 4-year follow-up.[42] Although this device requires additional study to assess its effectiveness compared with standard antireflux surgery and medical management, it does seem like an encouraging treatment option for elderly reflux patients who are unable or unwilling to go through the full fundoplication procedure.

Other surgical alternatives can have similar niche applications in the elderly reflux patient. Radiofrequency energy (ablation) delivered at the level of the LES is thought to produce muscle hypertrophy and improved competence of the valve. This treatment, known as *Stretta* (Mederi Therapeutics, Norwalk, CT, USA), is indicated for patients with refractory GERD, but was initially plagued with reports that the treatment does not produce significant changes, compared with sham therapy, in physiologic parameters, including duration of esophageal pH less than 4, ability to come off PPI therapy, or patient-reported quality of life.[43] Nonetheless, radiofrequency ablation therapy is regaining popularity in treating refractory reflux patients because of refinement of surgical protocol and improved patient selection. *EsophyX* (Endogastric Solutions, Redwood City, WA, USA) is a device reported to create an incisionless fundoplication. The device is placed transesophageally into the proximal gastric cavity, and a retroflexed stapler creates an internal "pexy" of the LES. Long-term data are not yet available for *EsophyX*. In short-term follow-up, from 6 months to 2 years, *EsophyX* may be most effective in patients with moderate to severe hiatal hernias.[44] Although unlikely to be a replacement for standard treatment options, attention should be given to the gastroenterology and general surgery literature in the coming years to evaluate which of these surgical alternatives may have a role in the treatment of the elderly reflux patient.

REFERENCES

1. Koufman JA, Aviv JE, Casiano RR, et al. Laryngopharyngeal reflux: position statement of the committee on speech, voice, and swallowing disorders of the American Academy of Otolaryngology-Head and Neck Surgery. Otolaryngol Head Neck Surg 2002;127(1):32–5.
2. Francis DO, Patel DA, Sharda R, et al. Patient-reported outcome measures related to laryngopharyngeal reflux: a systematic review of instrument development and validation. Otolaryngol Head Neck Surg 2016;155(6):923–35.
3. Belafsky PC, Postma GN, Koufman JA. Validity and reliability of the reflux symptom index (RSI). J Voice 2002;16:274–7.
4. Sidhwa F, Moore A, Alligood E, et al. Diagnosis and treatment of the extraesophageal manifestations of gastroesophageal reflux disease. Ann Surg 2017;265(1):63–7.
5. Patel D, Vaezi MF. Normal esophageal physiology and laryngopharyngeal reflux. Otolaryngol Clin North Am 2013;46(6):1023–41.
6. Fenter TC, Naslund MJ, Shah MB, et al. The cost of treating the 10 most prevalent diseases in men 50 years of age or older. Am J Manag Care 2006;12(4 Suppl):S90–8.
7. Everhart JE, Ruhl CE. Burden of digestive diseases in the United States part I: overall and upper gastrointestinal diseases. Gastroenterology 2009;136(2):376–86.

8. Francis DO, Rymer JA, Slaughter JC, et al. High economic burden of caring for patients with suspected extraesophageal reflux. Am J Gastroenterol 2013; 108(6):905–11.

9. Bureau UC. An aging world: 2015. Available at: https://www.census.gov/library/publications/2016/demo/P95-16-1.html. Accessed September 15, 2017.

10. Pilotto A, Maggi S, Noale M, et al. Association of upper gastrointestinal symptoms with functional and clinical charateristics in elderly. World J Gastroenterol 2011; 17(25):3020–6.

11. Pilotto A, Franceschi M, Leandro G, et al. Clinical features of reflux esophagitis in older people: a study of 840 consecutive patients. J Am Geriatr Soc 2006;54: 1537–42.

12. Barczi SR, Sullivan PA, Robbins J. How should dysphagia care of older adults differ? Establishing optimal practice patterns. Semin Speech Lang 2000;21: 347–61.

13. Collen MJ, Abdulian JD, Chen YK. Gastroesophageal reflux disease in the elderly: more severe disease that require aggressive therapy. Am J Gastroenterol 1995;90:1053–7.

14. Hollis JB, Castell DO. Esophageal function in elderly men. A new look at "presby-esophagus". Ann Intern Med 1974;91:897–904.

15. Hyun JJ, Bak Y-T. Clinical significance of hiatal hernia. Gut Liver 2011;5(3): 267–77.

16. Manes G, Pieramico O, Uomo G, et al. Relationship of sliding hiatus hernia to gastroesophageal reflux disease: a possible role for Helicobacter pylori infection? Dig Dis Sci 2003;48(2):303–7.

17. Ferriolli E, Oliveira RB, Matsuda NM, et al. Aging, esophageal motility, and gastro-esophageal reflux disease. J Am Geriatr Soc 1998;46:1534–7.

18. Sonnenberg A. Salivary secretion in reflux esophagitis. Gastroenterology 1982; 83:889–97.

19. Kawamura O, Aslam M, Rittmann T, et al. Physical and pH properties of gastro-esophagopharyngeal refluxate: a 24-hour simultaneous ambulatory impedance and pH monitoring study. Am J Gastroenterol 2004;99:1000–10.

20. Vaezi MF. Laryngitis and gastroesophageal reflux disease: increasing prevalence or poor diagnostic tests? Am J Gastroenterol 2004;99:786–8.

21. Steward DL, Wilson KM, Kelly DH, et al. Proton pump inhibitor therapy for chronic laryngopharyngitis: a randomized placebo-control trial. Otolaryngol Head Neck Surg 2004;131:342–50.

22. McGlashan JA, Johnstone LM, Sykes J, et al. The value of a liquid alginate suspension (Gaviscon Advance) in the management of laryngopharyngeal reflux. Eur Arch Otorhinolaryngol 2009;266(2):243–51.

23. Reichel O, Dressel H, Wiederanders K, et al. Double-blind, placebo-controlled trial with esomeprazole for symptoms and signs associated with laryngopharyng-eal reflux. Otolaryngol Head Neck Surg 2008;139(3):414–20.

24. Fass R, Noelck N, Willis MR, et al. The effect of esomeprazole 20 mg twice daily on acoustic and perception parameters of the voice in laryngopharyngeal reflux. Neurogastroenterol Motil 2010;22(2):134–41.

25. Haenisch B, von Holt K, Wiese B, et al. Risk of dementia in elderly patients with the use of proton pump inhibitors. Eur Arch Psychiatry Clin Neurosci 2015;265: 419–28.

26. Gomm W, von Holt K, Thome F, et al. Association between proton pump inhibitors with risk of dementia: a pharmacoepidemiological claims data analysis. JAMA Neurol 2016;73:410–6.

27. Taipale H, Tolppanen A-M, Tiihonen M, et al. No association between proton pump inhibitor use and risk of Alzheimer's disease. Am J Gastroenterol 2017; 112(12):1802–8.
28. Goldstein FC, Steenland K, Zhao L, et al. Proton pump inhibitors and risk of mild cognitive impairment and dementia. J Am Geriatr Soc 2017;65(9):1532–54.
29. Booker A, Jacob LE, Rapp M, et al. Risk factors for dementia diagnosis in German primary care practices. Int Psychogeriatr 2016;28(7):1059–65.
30. Moore AR, O'Keefe ST. Drug-induced cognitive impairment in the elderly. Drugs Aging 1999;15(1):15–28.
31. Fackler WK, Ours TM, Vaezi MF, et al. Long-term effect of H2RA therapy on nocturnal gastric acid breakthrough. Gastroenterology 2002;122:625–32.
32. de Caestecker J. Prokinetics and reflux: a promise unfulfilled. Eur J Gastroenterol Hepatol 2002;14:5–7.
33. Kahrilas PJ, Quigley EM, Castell DO, et al. The effects of tegaserod (HTF 919) on oesophageal acid exposure in gastro-oesophageal reflux disease. Aliment Pharmacol Ther 2000;14:1503–9.
34. Maret-Ouda J, Brusselaers N, Lagergren J. What is the most effective treatment for severe gastro-oesophageal reflux disease? BMJ 2015;350:h3169.
35. Lundell L, Attwood S, Ell C, et al, LOTUS Trial Collaborators. Comparing laparoscopic antireflux surgery with esomeprazole in the management of patients with chronic gastro-oesophageal reflux disease: a 3-year interim analysis of the LOTUS trial. Gut 2008;57(9):1207–13.
36. Grant AM, Boachie C, Cotton SC, et al, REFLUX Trial Group. Clinical and economic evaluation of laparoscopic surgery compared with medical management for gastro-oesophageal reflux disease: 5-year follow-up of multicentre randomised trial (the REFLUX trial). Health Technol Assess 2013;17(22):1–167.
37. Anvari M, Allen C, Marshall J, et al. A randomized controlled trial of laparoscopic Nissen fundoplication versus proton pump inhibitors for the treatment of patients with chronic gastroesophageal reflux disease (GERD): 3-year outcomes. Surg Endosc 2011;25(8):2547–54.
38. Maret-Ouda J, Wahlin K, El-Serag HB, et al. Association between laparoscopic antireflux surgery and recurrence of gastroesophageal reflux. JAMA 2017; 318(10):939–46.
39. Fei L, Rossetti G, Moccia F, et al. Is the advanced age a contraindication to GERD laparoscopic surgery? Results of a long term follow-up. BMC Surg 2013;13(suppl 2):S13.
40. Morgenthal CB, Lin E, Shane MD, et al. Who will fail laparoscopic Nissen fundoplication? Preoperative prediction of long-term outcomes. Surg Endosc 2007; 21(11):1978–84.
41. Dallemagne B, Arenas Sanchez M, Francart D, et al. Long-term results after laparoscopic reoperation for failed antireflux procedures. Br J Surg 2011;98(11): 1581–7.
42. Lipham JC, DeMeester TR, Ganz RA, et al. The LINX reflux management system: confirmed safety and efficacy now at 4 years. Surg Endosc 2012;26(10):2944–9.
43. Lipka S, Kumar A, Richter JE. No evidence for efficacy of radiofrequency ablation for treatment of gastroesophageal reflux disease: a systematic review and meta-analysis. Clin Gastroenterol Hepatol 2015;13(6):1058–67.e1.
44. Auyang ED, Carter P, Rauth T, et al. SAGES clinical spotlight review: endoluminal treatments for gastroesophageal reflux disease (GERD). Surg Endosc 2013; 27(8):2658–72.

Facial Plastic Surgery in the Geriatric Population

Ian Newberry, MD[a], Eric W. Cerrati, MD[a,*], J. Regan Thomas, MD[b]

KEYWORDS

- Aging face • Facial rejuvenation • Brow-ptosis • Dermatochalasis • Jowls

KEY POINTS

- Geriatric facial rejuvenation is an elective procedure that requires a thorough preoperative assessment to circumvent perioperative complications.
- Facial aging is an inevitable process that largely results from soft tissue descent and volumetric deflation.
- A comprehensive knowledge of the aging process and precise assessment of the exact pathologies yielding the patient's appearance is essential to produce the best cosmetic outcome.
- In the aging population, minimally invasive procedures alone are often insufficient to address the excessive skin laxity. A combination of surgical and nonsurgical interventions often yields the best cosmetic result.
- The aging face must be evaluated as a whole to reduce the unnatural appearance seen when regions are addressed independently.

INTRODUCTION

Greater life expectancy with advancements in technology and medicine has lead to a growing interest in management of the aging process. In particular, concern with facial rejuvenation has dramatically expanded in both the medical and societal realms. The face is vital to the idea of beauty and plays a principle role in human perception with studies showing that attractive people make more money and are considered more "able" by employers. With the growing geriatric population, the media's portrayal of elegant aging and ideal image, the advent of social media, and the reduction of stigma surrounding cosmetic surgery, the pursuit of youthful appearance for personal and professional reasons has become the cornerstone in the fastest growing medical sector.[1,2]

Disclosure: The authors have nothing to disclose.
[a] Facial Plastic and Reconstructive Surgery, Division of Otolaryngology–Head and Neck Surgery, University of Utah, 30 No. 1900 East Room 3C120 SOM, Salt Lake City, Utah 84132, USA;
[b] Division of Facial Plastic and Reconstructive Surgery, Department of Otolaryngology-Head and Neck Surgery, Northwestern University, NMH/Arkes Family Pavilion Suite 1325, 676 N Saint Clair, Chicago, IL 60611, USA
* Corresponding author.
E-mail address: eric.cerrati@hsc.utah.edu

Otolaryngol Clin N Am 51 (2018) 789–802
https://doi.org/10.1016/j.otc.2018.03.013
0030-6665/18/© 2018 Elsevier Inc. All rights reserved.

Preoperative Evaluation

First and foremost, the surgeon must appreciate the elective nature of facial rejuvenation, because many of the techniques require a trip to the operating room and general anesthesia. During the initial surgical evaluation, it is important to be cognizant of patient's comorbidities, functional status, and medications. Preoperative assessment and medical clearance by a primary care physician is often necessary as well as preoperative anesthesia consultation and possible cardiology clearance in higher risk patients.

The Aging Process

A comprehensive knowledge of the aging process and precise assessment of the exact pathologies yielding the patient's appearance is essential to achieve the best cosmetic outcome. Facial aging is an inevitable process that largely results from soft tissue descent and volumetric deflation. The main elements of facial anatomy are skin, muscles, ligaments, fat, and the bony skeleton. During the aging process, skin becomes inelastic, coarse, saggy, and dyschromic. Diffuse lipoatrophy causes facial hollowing and the potential laxity of facial retaining ligaments allows for descent or pseudoherniation of atrophied fat pads, making orbital and nasolabial fat pads as well as jowls more prominent.[3,4] Mimetic muscles undergo sarcopenia and increase in tone to near maximal contracture character contributing to wrinkle formation. Further, the facial skeleton undergoes heterogeneous reabsorption. Regions with strong predisposition for resorption include the midface, the superomedial and inferolateral orbital rim, the prejowl area of the mandible, and the alveolar ridges.[5–7] This bony resorption contributes to prominent upper lid medial fat pads, deepening of the nasojugal groove, flat and hollowed cheeks, and deepening of the geniomandibular groove exaggerating jowl appearance.[8] The facial plastic surgeon must keep in mind that, in addition to tightening and resurfacing procedures, cosmetic outcomes might improve when volumetric reduction is addressed.[5,9]

Skin

Aging skin is one of the primary characteristics of the aging face and must be addressed as a part of comprehensive facial rejuvenation. Senescent skin changes occur owing to both intrinsic and extrinsic aging. Intrinsic aging occurs when proliferation slows and the number of epidermal cells decrease.[10] Collagen, elastic fibers, and glycosaminoglycans, particularly hyaluronic acid, are reduced secondary to decreased synthesis and a slight increase in degradatory matrix metalloproteinases.[11] Together, these processes can result in fine static rhytids and inelastic, thin-appearing skin that may exaggerate dynamic wrinkling. However, the most dramatic effects are secondary to extrinsic factors, such as ultraviolet radiation and smoking. In extrinsic aging, photoaging secondary to ultraviolet radiation is the largest culprit. Shorter wavelength ultraviolet B light primarily penetrates the epidermis to elicit keratinocytic and melanocytic damage, while longer wavelength ultraviolet A light penetrates into the dermis. Photoaging leads to a profound dermal collagen decrease and degradation as well as elastosis—dermal accumulation of disorganized elastic fibers and glycosaminoglycans.[11] These effects lead to exaggerated static rhytids, deep furrows, elastosis with thickened, sallow, coarse-appearing skin, telangiectasias, and areas of dyschromia.

In managing senescent skin changes, the prevention of extrinsic damage plays a crucial role. Long-term medical therapy with topical medications is vital in the management and prevention of aging skin. Topical retinoids improve the appearance of mild to moderate photodamage (fine to course wrinkles, roughness, pigmentation) through the regulation of gene expression to increase procollagen.[12] Hydroxyl acids (glycolic acid, lactic acid, salicylic acid) encourage exfoliation and skin cell turnover, but primarily improve dyspigmentation and roughness, rather than fine wrinkles.[13]

Once aging has developed, careful selection of treatment is based on patient skin type and degree of photoaging. The Glogau classification system provides an assessment to categorize and guide possible treatment (**Table 1**).[14,15] Patients with mild photoaging can often be managed conservatively with superficial peels and lasers, microdermabrasion, and proper skin care. Patients with moderate photoaging can be managed with medium-depth peels in addition to long-term medical therapy. Advanced to severe photoaging will usually require medium to deep chemical peels, ablative lasers, or dermabrasion with a long-term medical therapy.

Dermabrasion can best aid in the rejuvenation of moderate to severe rhytids, especially in the perioral regions. Laser use is steadily increasing and is best used for moderate to severe photodamage. The primary lasers used for facial resurfacing are the pulsed CO_2 and Er:YAG, which are particularly useful for static rhytids, diffuse coarseness, and dyschromias. Resurfacing procedures all work similarly by removing the epidermis and damaging varying degrees of dermis to bring about a fresh layer of skin and stimulate elastotic fiber regeneration and procollagen production.[14] Notably, although folds and deep furrows in dynamic wrinkle zones may be improved with resurfacing, particular tightening surgeries in addition to botulinum toxin and filler injections may be required to manage the aging face and are discussed by region herein.

The Upper One-Third of the Face

Forehead and temple

The forehead and temple play a major role in supporting and framing the upper brow, lateral orbital rim, and upper eyelid. The forehead occupies the central three-fifths of the upper face, and is delineated by the (1) hairline superiorly, (2) temporal ridge laterally, (3) and supraorbital ridge and glabella inferiorly. The temples occupy the other lateral fifths.

The aging forehead appearance is predominantly owing to the formation of deep static furrows from the cumulative effect of muscle's repetitive firing and contracture in combination with senescent skin changes.[16] The rhytids will form primarily perpendicular to the orientation of the underlying mimetic muscles.[2] The frontalis muscles, the primary brow elevators, produce the several long horizontal forehead rhytids. The corrugator supercillii muscle has 2 heads that adduct and depress the medial

Table 1		
Glogau scale for severity of photoaging		
Classification	**Rhytid Description**	**Skin Description**
Group I (mild)	Absent to little wrinkles	Minimal to no wrinkles, mild pigmentary changes, and no kerotoses or solar lentigines
Group II (moderate)	Wrinkles in motion	Obvious dynamic wrinkles, mild fine static wrinkles, pigmentary changes with faint senile lentigines (brown spots)
Group III (advanced)	Wrinkles at rest	Prominent static wrinkles or furrows, apparent dyschromia, visible actinic keratosis, telangiectasias, solar lentigines
Group IV (severe)	Wrinkles throughout	Deep static wrinkles throughout, coarse, thickened, sallow skin, diffuse kerotoses, prior skin malignancies, no normal skin

brow, generating the frowned appearance, and is the principal source of vertical and oblique glabellar lines. Its depth must be considered during botulinum injections. After originating near the medial supraorbital rim, the corrugator courses deep to the depressor supercilii and orbicularis muscles as it primarily runs transversely to become more superficial and interdigitate with the frontalis over the midbrow.[17] The unpaired procerus muscle arises from the nasal bones then runs vertically to insert in the dermis, producing transverse glabellar rhytids.

With forehead aging, there is also the formation of true brow ptosis owing to gravitational forces, collagen and elastin defects, action of brow depressors, and soft tissue–bony volume loss in the brow–temporal region. In the treatment of mild brow ptosis, botulinum injection into the superotemporal orbicularis oculi muscle can give a modest 1 to 2 mm lateral lift, and filler injections can deliver some brow augmentation by providing slight brow elevation as well as decreasing the pseudoptosis effects of upper lid and temporal hollowing.[18,19]

The temple regions are convexly shaped areas that softly blend into the lateral orbital rim, zygomatic arch, and temporal line. With lipoatrophy and temporal muscle wasting, the region takes on a sunken, emaciated appearance that increases the prominence of the temporal orbital rim, temporal line, and inferior zygomatic arch, as well as contributes to lateral brow ptosis. Biostimulatory fillers that promote collagen formation such ploy-L-lactic acid (Sculptra; Galderma, Lausanne, Switzerland), and calcium hydroxyapatitie (Radiesse; Merz Aesthetic, Frankfurt, Germany) or hyaluronic acid can be injected to augment the hollowed appearance and gently elevate the tail of the brow.[18,20]

In summary, treatment of the aging forehead can be managed with botulinum injections, filler instillations, lasers, or surgical procedures; however, depending on the particular patient, a combination of techniques may offer the best cosmetic rejuvenation (**Fig. 1**).[16,18,19]

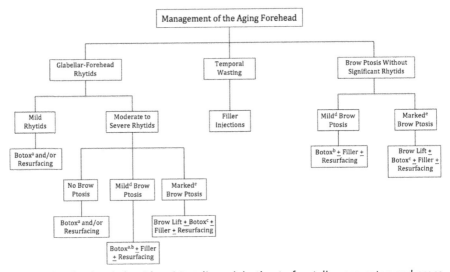

Fig. 1. Aging forehead algorithm. [a] Botulinum injection to frontalis, corrugator, and procerus. [b] Botulinum to the superotemporal orbicularis occuli while ensuring the injections do not extend to the very lateral or inferior frontalis. [c] After a brow lift, botulinum injection in solely the brow depressors during the healing process has been shown to improve longevity and cosmetic result. [d] Mild ptosis (<2 mm). [e] Marked ptosis (>3 mm).

The brow–eyelid continuum

Periorbital aging can manifest as brow ptosis, dermatochalasis (true eyelid redundancy and laxity), rhytids, steatoblepharon (orbital fat herniation), or contour irregularities owing to orbital rim resorption and lipoatrophy.

It is important to avoid the assessment of the forehead, brow, or eyelid in isolation, but rather as a continuum that influences one another. A common complaint, droopy upper eyelids, can be due to brow ptosis shifting infrabrow skin inferiorly (pseudodermatochalasis), dermatochalasis, steatoblepharon, or, frequently, a combination of processes.[21,22] If blepharoplasty is performed without the recognition of underlying brow ptosis, poor cosmesis may result because the subsequent narrowed brow–lid margin pulls the brow further inferiorly. Alternatively, if the patient had unrecognized chronic frontalis activation trying to elevate the redundant eyelid skin, the removal of skin may unmask brow ptosis and allow the reappearance of inferiorly shifted skin as the drive for frontalis activation is diminished.

When assessing the brow, familiarity with the ideal brow is essential: (1) the brow originates vertical of medial canthus and roughly terminates at a point on a line drawn from the alar base through the lateral canthus, (2) the medial and lateral ends lie almost on the same horizontal plane, (3) the female brow should lie at or slightly below orbital rim medially then gently arch laterally above the rim with the apex roughly 1 cm above the rim just medial to the lateral canthus, and (4) the male brow should be at or slightly below rim with a more horizontal orientation.[22,23] Relaxation of the frontalis muscle must be confirmed; then, the degree of brow elevation required from the ptotic position should be recorded. The primary region of ptosis will be the lateral brow.[24] During the consultation, the brow should be stabilized into a natural or ideal position to allow for the proper evaluation of the upper lid. Mild ptosis may be managed with botulinum toxin and fillers (see **Fig. 1**), whereas marked ptosis requires a surgical brow lift. Several variables are factored into choosing the appropriate brow lift technique, such as location of the hairline, hairstyle of the patient, and the presence of asymmetry (**Table 2**). For all these techniques, it is critically important to fully release the periosteum at the superior orbital rim to achieve the desired lift that will be maintained over time. Blepharoplasty techniques may then be used to excise redundant skin and redistribute or remove orbital fat.

When evaluating the periorbital rejuvenation patient, the surgeon must also rule out blepharoptosis (low eyelid margin) or pseudoblepharoptosis owing to eyelid redundancy. With age, the levator aponeurosis can become stretched, dehiscent, or disinserted from the tarsal plate causing aponeurotic blepharoptosis.[25] The normal upper eyelid margin should fall approximately 1 to 2 mm below the superior limbus and have a marginal reflex distance of 4 mm or more.[22] Common methods of blepharoptosis repair are levator palpebrae advancement or Muller muscle resection.[25]

The Middle One-Third of the Face

Lower eyelid

Often, the earliest periorbital aging sign is the development of rhytids near the lateral canthi, known as crow's feet. As aging proceeds, skin and orbicularis laxity progresses and the orbital septum weakens enabling fat pseudoherniation to produce the characteristic lower eyelid bags.

The fundamental considerations with lower lid blepharoplasty are the (1) degree of orbital fat prolapse, (2) magnitude of lid redundancy, (3) degree of infraorbital hallowing, and (4) lower lid laxity. Patients who predominantly have an abundance of fat herniation can undergo the transconjunctival approach for the excision and redraping of the fat pads. In the older population, this approach often has to be coupled with a skin

Table 2		
Comparison of various brow lifting procedures		
Advantages and Disadvantages of Various Forehead and Brow Lifts		
Procedure	Advantages	Disadvantages
Chemical (nonsurgical) brow lift (Botox with or without filler injections with or without resurfacing)	• No surgical procedure required • May help those with very mild brow ptosis	• Can elevate brows only 1–2 mm, potentially more if multiple nonsurgical interventions • Results are temporary (3–5 mo)
Browpexy (transblepharoplasty)	• May help with mild brow ptosis • May help in females with minimal ptosis causing a flatter, androgynous eyebrow appearance • More minimally invasive procedure with a single incision if upper blepharoplasty is also indicated	• Does not address forehead/glabellar rhytids • Some have found this to be somewhat unreliable, unpredictable, short lived • Cannot repair severe brow ptosis • Possible prolonged eyelid anesthesia and edema
Endoscopic brow lift	• More minimally invasive procedure, faster recovery • Reduced scaring compared with open procedures • Treats most aspects of upper face aging including glabellar/forehead rhytids and brow ptosis	• Slight-to-moderate elevation of hairline • Contour irregularities of scalp • Degree of brow elevation may not be as much as open procedures
Bilateral temporal lift (open or endoscopic)	• Addresses temporal brow ptosis • Does not alter central hairline, no central scar. • Can be used in male pattern baldness.	• No effect on medial brow • Does not address midforehead/glabellar rhytids
Midforehead brow lift	• No hairline elevation. Best in males with prominent forehead rhytids and receding hairline/baldness • Can address glabellar rhytids • More functional than cosmetic; can be used in facial paralysis and patients not concerned with scaring • Better correction of asymmetry	• Lowers hairline • Prominent forehead scar; may be better hidden in forehead furrows • Significant lateral brow elevation is difficult to achieve
Direct brow lift	• More functional than cosmetic; can be used in facial paralysis and patients not concerned with scaring • Quick procedure that can performed under local in those with extensive comorbidities • More precise brow elevation and correction of asymmetry	• Feminizes the brow as feathered superior edge hairs are lost giving a manicured look • Possible visible scar; best hid in those with bushy, dark-colored eyebrows
Trichophytic forehead lift	• Maintains or lowers hairline; men without baldness, women with a high hairline, large forehead	• Possible visible scaring • Prominent scarring if hairline recedes

(continued on next page)

Table 2
(*continued*)

Advantages and Disadvantages of Various Forehead and Brow Lifts		
Procedure	Advantages	Disadvantages
	• Treats most aspects of upper face aging, including glabellar/forehead rhytids and brow ptosis	• Possible prolonged scalp hypesthesia • Less precise brow elevation
Coronal forehead lift	• Treats most aspects of upper face aging including glabellar/forehead rhytids and brow ptosis • Can be used if low hairline, small forehead	• Elevates hairline and lengthens forehead • Possible prolonged scalp hypesthesia • Prominent scarring if balding ensues • Less precise brow elevation

pinch excision to address the excess lower lid skin. More commonly, a transcutaneous (eg, subciliary) approach is better able to address the excess skin, excess orbicularis muscle, and fat herniation. If a tear trough deformity is present, fat transposition can be used. Another common finding in the aging population is lower lid laxity, lid malposition (entropion, ectropion), and/or increased scleral show. For these patients, lower lid tightening maneuvers should be performed and can include a canthopexy, a tarsal strip, or a muscle suspension.

Midface and nasaolabial region

An important youthful characteristic is the fullness of the upper midface relative to the flatter lower portion. On three-quarter and profile inspection, the maximal area of volume is located in a single upper convexity, formed by the suborbicularis oculi fat (SOOF) and malar fat pad, then transitions into a mild concavity at the inferior aspect of the cheek. This S-shaped curve is called the midface ogee curve.[19] With deflation and descent of the SOOF, orbicularis oculi, and malar fat, a double convexity deformity results with a disrupted ogee curve (**Fig. 2**). The lower eyelid bags form the upper convexity while the lower convexity is formed by the descended SOOF, malar fat, and orbicularis.[26] The depression between the 2 convexities is formed between the orbitomalar and zygomatic retaining ligaments. Tissue and edema can accumulate in this valley to develop bulges called malar bags or festoons (see **Fig. 2**).[19]

Midface ptosis also allows for the accumulation of malar soft tissue adjacent to the nasolabial fold, accounting for its prominence with aging, as well as contributes to the formation of the tear trough deformity (nasojugal groove) and jowling. An important midface retaining ligament is the orbital retaining (orbitalmalar) ligament. Possible relaxation of this ligament contributes to the orbicularis muscle and SOOF descent and to the nasojugal groove, explaining the importance of sufficiently releasing the orbitalmalar ligament during lifting procedures.

The goal of midface surgery is the elevation of the malar soft tissues and directed midface revolumization to accomplish the following: (1) decreased nasolabial appearance, (2) cheek projection, (3) reestablished ogee curve, and (4) diminished nasojugal grooves, but can also (5) improve the aged lower face–neck appearance.[27]

Mild midface ptosis can be repaired through a lower blepharoplasty approach. By releasing the orbitalmalar ligament, the SOOF can be identified, elevated, and resuspended onto the orbital rim to improve lid–cheek contour and the nasojugal groove. Another option for midface elevation is a deep plane facelift. The superficial muscular

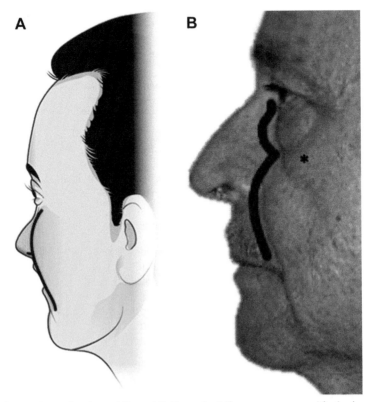

Fig. 2. Comparison of aging midface. (*A*) Normal midface ogee curve with single convexity over malar eminence. (*B*) Aging midface with double convexity deformity. The lower midface may continue to flatten. (*Asterisk*) Malar mound and festoon.

aponeurotic system imbrication or plication rhytidectomy (facelift) is best used to treat the neck and jowls rather than the nasolabial fold; however, for mild midface ptosis and lower face–neck aging, SMAS rhytidectomy is particularly helpful. For more marked midface ptosis, especially with significant nasolabial folds and jowling, a deep-plane (sub-SMAS) rhytidectomy may be required to ensure the retaining ligaments (eg, zygomatic and mandibular ligaments) are released. Recent anatomic studies have shown a lack of SMAS attachment to the nasolabial folds.[28] With the risks of subperiosteal and deep approaches, some surgeons elect for SMAS facelifts with directed revolumization to the malar prominence, nasolabial folds, or nasojugal groove to disguise the aged appearance.

Nose
With age, the supporting structures of the nose weaken to affect both esthetics and function. Visually, the most notable change is the apparent lengthening of the nose with tip ptosis, which may give a pseudo-dorsal hump appearance.[2] Cosmetic changes are primarily owing to weakening of the lower lateral cartilages, anterior nasal spine resorption with retraction of the columella, interdomal ligament attenuation, and weakening of the scroll's fibroelastic connections leading to downward migration of lateral cura.[29] Columellar strut grafts, tip grafts, and various suture techniques (eg,

tongue-in-groove maneuver, transdomal or interdomal sutures) can be used to increase tip support, projection, and rotation, improving the aged appearance.[30]

With tip ptosis, inferior turbinate hypertrophy, and separation of upper and lower lateral cura, internal nasal valve collapse is common among the elderly. In addition to addressing tip ptosis, septorhinoplasty, turbinate reduction, and grafts (eg, spreader grafts) are used to address internal nasal valve collapse.[2,30] External nasal valve collapse is also common owing to weakened lower lateral cartilages.

The Lower Face

Perioral region

Aging of the perioral region is characterized by vertical perioral rhytids radiating from the vermilion border, downturned oral commissures, marionette lines (labiomandibular folds), thin, elongated and flat upper lips, and thin, inverted lower lips. Lips will have poor architecture with diminished vermillion borders as well as thin red lip (vermillion) portions owing to muscle and fat atrophy. In particular, the upper lip will have flattening of its 2 high vermillion points (Cupid's bow), elongation of its cutaneous (white) lip leading to an inverted and thin appearing red lip, and loss of its bilateral philtrum columns and normal central concavity (**Fig. 3**).

Various surgical and nonsurgical procedures can be used to augment the perioral region. A lip lift, an elliptical excision of infranasal skin at the base of the nose, can give lasting results with increased visible red lip, a more pleasant and everted shape, and shorter cutaneous lip length.[2,19] To nonsurgically enhance the lip's architecture, an injectable filler (hyaluronic acid) is injected along the white line (rolled borders), philtrum, and Cupid's bow. To address the volume, the injection is along the lip's vermillion body, just anterior to wet–dry border.[18,31] Volumizing the marionette folds along with botulinum injections into the depressor anguli oris can help to improve the downward posture of the oral commissures and decrease labiomandibular folds.[18] Again, for deeper, static rhytids, resurfacing procedures and injectable fillers are used whereas dynamic or very fine rhytids can be aided by resurfacing or botulinum injections.

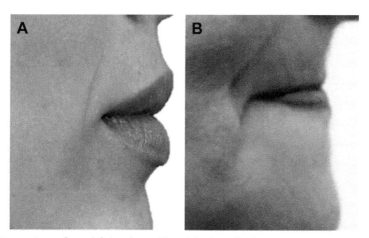

Fig. 3. Comparison of youthful and aged lips. (A) In youth, the cutaneous lip is concave and shorter with curvaceous, volumized vermillion lips to give the attractive "pouty" appearance. (B) The senescent cutaneous lip is elongated, flatter, and almost convex with inverted, thin vermillion lips.

Table 3
Targeted management of the lower face and neck based on particular pathologies highlighted within Dedo's classification

Dedo's Classification	Description	Targeted Lower Face–Cervical Treatment Plan		
		Illustration	Primary Intervention	Supplemental Treatment
Class I (mild deformity)	Defined cervicomental angle (90°–120°), minimal fat, good skin and platysmal tone		• No surgical intervention • Prophylactic limited rhytidectomy (eg, S-lift) • Resurfacing	• With or without chin implant (micrognathia) • With or without osteotomies (retrognathia) • With or without filler injections
Class II (skin)	Excessive skin laxity contributing to jowling, horizontal cervical rhytids, and effaced cervicomental angle		• Rhytidectomy (face lift of lower face and neck)	• With or without cervical liposuction if ptotic jowl fat or submental fat • With or without anterior platysmaplasty for dehiscent, lax platysma • With or without chin implant
Class III (fat)	Excessive fat accumulation in the supraplatysmal or subplatysmal plane or ptotic fat		• Direct removal or cervical liposuction targeting submental compartments for anterior neck fullness and ptotic jowl fat	• With or without anterior platysmaplasty for dehiscent, lax platysma • With or without chin implant • With or without rhytidectomy for skin laxity or redundancy

Class	Description		Treatment
Class IV (muscle)	Platysmal laxity and banding; apparent at rest in thin neck or may become apparent with contraction in thicker neck		• Anterior platysmaplasty with plication of medial borders, possible horizontal platysma incisions and excision of redundant medial platysma • Rhytidectomy as SMAS/platysma suspension tightens platysma and skin • With or without chin implant • With or without cervical liposuction for ptotic or excessive fat
Class V (bone)	Congenital/acquired micrognathia (underprojected chin) or deficient mandibular height or retrognathia (retruded mandible, class 2 occlusion)		• Chin augmentation with chin/ angle implants and fillers (micrognathia) • Osteotomy (retrognathia and deficient vertical mandibular height)
Class VI (bone-cartilage)	Abnormally low or anterior hyoid, short hyomental distance		• Treat concomitant abnormalities with understanding inability to fully correct irregularities • Possible division of suprahyoid musculature • Possible suturing the anterior digastrics together

Data from Dedo DD. "How I do it"–plastic surgery. Practical suggestions on facial plastic surgery. A preoperative classification of the neck for cervicofacial rhytidectomy. Laryngoscope 1980;90(11 Pt 1):1894–6.

Jawline and neck

Within the lower one-third of the face as well as the neck, a number of associated changes contribute to the aged appearance. First, factors that contribute to the youthful, attractive appearance include a (1) distinct cervicomental angle between 90 and 120° maintained by taut submental skin with minimal submental adipose tissue, a high posterior hyoid bone, and a strong mentum, (2) strong chin with its pogonion at or just anterior to a line drawn from the lower lip in men and at or slightly posterior in women, (3) distinct mandibular border demarcating the face–neck, (4) well-visualized thyroid cartilage, and (5) neck with distinct anterior sternocleidomastoid muscle borders, minimal skin folds, and no anterior platysmal neck bands.[19,32]

Jowl formation, one of the primary complaints of aging patients, interrupts a well-defined mandibular border. Jowls occur from the combination of premasseteric space ptosis, descent of superior and inferior jowl fat, increased skin laxity, submandibular gland ptosis, and reduced mandibular height.[4,33] A prejowl sulcus, formed as bone resorbs and tissue atrophies within the geniomandibular groove, and marionette lines may exaggerate the jowling appearance.[4,8] Although marionette lines are improved with facelifts, it may be critical to release the mandibular ligament to fully eliminate the lines. However, if the lines and sulcus remain after rhytidectomy or if the initial jowling is minimal, filler injections alone into this region may improve the appearance.[18]

With aging, dehiscence and excess laxity of the platysma in the anterior neck creates submental fullness and effacement of the cervicomental angle. With progression, prominent vertical bands in the anterior neck may form. The submandibular fat pad and glands then lose support and may become ptotic, furthering the submental fullness. Isolated or concomitant cervical–submental liposis, with accumulation of fat in the supraplatysmal or subplatysmal layer, can lead to cervical fullness. Finally, premental fat ptosis, deepening of the labiomental crease, and bony resorption leading to reduced mandibular height and projection all contribute to acquired micrognathia, which subsequently contributes to a weak chin appearance, increased cervicomental angle, and indistinct mandibular border.

The Dedo's preoperative classification can help to delineate a patient's specific pathology and help to guide targeted treatment (**Table 3**).[34] Although this classification is useful, many patients will have more than 1 class of deformity. In addition to the defects highlighted by Dedo's classification, ptotic submandibular glands can lead to submental fullness and limit cosmetic outcome. Many cosmetic surgeons hesitate to perform cosmetic submandibulectomy owing to the high risk of marginal mandibular, lingual, and hypoglossal nerve injury; however, SMAS rhytidectomy and platysmaplasty to plicate the dehiscent medial platysma borders can improve ptotic glands.[35] Despite the numerous procedures in the literature, the rhytidectomy (neck and face lift) remains one of the most powerful procedures to improve the appearance of the lower face and neck because it can soften marionette lines, decrease jowls, improve the cervicomental angle, define the mandibular border, reduce platysma laxity, and remove skin redundancies.[36] Last, although much can be done, poor anatomy (eg, inferior-anterior hyoid) and diffuse cervicofacial liposis can limit cosmetic outcomes and should be discussed preoperatively.

REFERENCES

1. Honigman R, Castle DJ. Aging and cosmetic enhancement. Clin Interv Aging 2006;1(2):115–9.

2. Friedman O. Changes associated with the aging face. Facial Plast Surg Clin North Am 2005;13(3):371–80.
3. Cotofana S, Fratila AA, Schenck TL, et al. The anatomy of the aging face: a review. Facial Plast Surg 2016;32(3):253–60.
4. Alghoul M, Codner MA. Retaining ligaments of the face: review of anatomy and clinical applications. Aesthet Surg J 2013;33(6):769–82.
5. Gerth DJ. Structural and volumetric changes in the aging face. Facial Plast Surg 2015;31(1):3–9.
6. Kahn DM, Shaw RB Jr. Aging of the bony orbit: a three-dimensional computed tomographic study. Aesthet Surg J 2008;28(3):258–64.
7. Ilankovan V. Anatomy of ageing face. Br J Oral Maxillofac Surg 2014;52(3):195–202.
8. Mendelson B, Wong CH. Changes in the facial skeleton with aging: implications and clinical applications in facial rejuvenation. Aesthetic Plast Surg 2012;36(4):753–60.
9. Little JW. Three-dimensional rejuvenation of the midface: volumetric resculpture by malar imbrication. Plast Reconstr Surg 2000;105(1):267–85 [discussion: 286–9].
10. Fenske NA, Lober CW. Structural and functional changes of normal aging skin. J Am Acad Dermatol 1986;15(4 Pt 1):571–85.
11. Naylor EC, Watson RE, Sherratt MJ. Molecular aspects of skin ageing. Maturitas 2011;69(3):249–56.
12. Samuel M, Brooke RC, Hollis S, et al. Interventions for photodamaged skin. Cochrane Database Syst Rev 2005;(1):CD001782.
13. Thomas JR, Dixon TK, Bhattacharyya TK. Effects of topicals on the aging skin process. Facial Plast Surg Clin North Am 2013;21(1):55–60.
14. Flint PW, Haughey BH, Robbins KT, et al. Cummings otolaryngology : head and neck surgery. 6th edition. London: Elsevier Health Sciences; 2015.
15. Durai PC, Thappa DM, Kumari R, et al. Aging in elderly: chronological versus photoaging. Indian J Dermatol 2012;57(5):343–52.
16. Fitzgerald R. Contemporary concepts in brow and eyelid aging. Clin Plast Surg 2013;40(1):21–42.
17. Beer JI, Sieber DA, Scheuer JF 3rd, et al. Three-dimensional facial anatomy: structure and function as it relates to injectable neuromodulators and soft tissue fillers. Plast Reconstr Surg Glob Open 2016;4(12 Suppl Anatomy and Safety in Cosmetic Medicine: Cosmetic Bootcamp):e1175.
18. Greco TM, Antunes MB, Yellin SA. Injectable fillers for volume replacement in the aging face. Facial Plast Surg 2012;28(1):8–20.
19. Ko AC, Korn BS, Kikkawa DO. The aging face. Surv Ophthalmol 2017;62(2): 190–202.
20. Misiek DJ, Kent JN, Carr RF. Soft tissue responses to hydroxylapatite particles of different shapes. J Oral Maxillofac Surg 1984;42(3):150–60.
21. Czyz CN, Hill RH, Foster JA. Preoperative evaluation of the brow-lid continuum. Clin Plast Surg 2013;40(1):43–53.
22. Lam VB, Czyz CN, Wulc AE. The brow-eyelid continuum: an anatomic perspective. Clin Plast Surg 2013;40(1):1–19.
23. Sclafani AP, Jung M. Desired position, shape, and dynamic range of the normal adult eyebrow. Arch Facial Plast Surg 2010;12(2):123–7.
24. Matros E, Garcia JA, Yaremchuk MJ. Changes in eyebrow position and shape with aging. Plast Reconstr Surg 2009;124(4):1296–301.
25. Wada Y, Hashimoto T, Kakizaki H, et al. What is the best way to handle the involutional blepharoptosis repair? J Craniofac Surg 2015;26(5):e377–80.
26. McCann JD, Pariseau B. Lower eyelid and midface rejuvenation. Facial Plast Surg 2013;29(4):273–80.

27. Jacono AA, Rousso JJ. An algorithmic approach to multimodality midfacial rejuvenation using a new classification system for midfacial aging. Clin Plast Surg 2015;42(1):17–32.

28. Buchanan DR, Wulc AE. Contemporary thoughts on lower eyelid/midface aging. Clin Plast Surg 2015;42(1):1–15.

29. Truswell WHT. Aging changes of the periorbita, cheeks, and midface. Facial Plast Surg 2013;29(1):3–12.

30. Rohrich RJ, Hollier LH Jr, Janis JE, et al. Rhinoplasty with advancing age. Plast Reconstr Surg 2004;114(7):1936–44.

31. Luthra A. Shaping lips with fillers. J Cutan Aesthet Surg 2015;8(3):139–42.

32. Patel BC. Aesthetic surgery of the aging neck: options and techniques. Orbit 2006;25(4):327–56.

33. Reece EM, Pessa JE, Rohrich RJ. The mandibular septum: anatomical observations of the jowls in aging-implications for facial rejuvenation. Plast Reconstr Surg 2008;121(4):1414–20.

34. Dedo DD. "How I do it" –plastic surgery. Practical suggestions on facial plastic surgery. A preoperative classification of the neck for cervicofacial rhytidectomy. Laryngoscope 1980;90(11 Pt 1):1894–6.

35. Lukavsky R, Linkov G, Fundakowski C. A novel approach to submandibular gland ptosis: creation of a platysma muscle and hyoid bone cradle. Arch Plast Surg 2016;43(4):374–8.

36. Sykes JM. Rejuvenation of the aging neck. Facial Plast Surg 2001;17(2):99–107.

Rhinitis and Sinusitis in the Geriatric Population

David W. Hsu, MD, Jeffrey D. Suh, MD*

KEYWORDS

- Allergic rhinitis • Nonallergic rhinitis • Acute rhinosinusitis
- Chronic rhinosinusitis without polyposis • Chronic rhinosinusitis with polyposis

KEY POINTS

- Changes in nasal anatomy and function in the elderly include decreased mucociliary clearance, decrease in immune function, and structural changes, which in turn lead to paranasal sinus disease.
- The geriatric population suffers from both allergic and nonallergic rhinitis, and both require specific pharmacotherapy in the setting of comorbidities and polypharmacy.
- Signs and symptoms of rhinitis may represent systemic, neoplastic, or other processes.
- Chronic rhinosinusitis in the elderly population may be unique in its pathogenesis in terms of host and microbial factors, but management is overall similar to the adult population.

INTRODUCTION

Rhinitis and sinusitis are among the most common medical conditions and are frequently associated. Rhinosinusitis can significantly affect a patient's quality of life (QOL), resulting in decreased productivity, poor sleep quality, and depression.[1,2] The geriatric population is increasing in the United States, representing 20% of the population.[3] According to the 2014 US Census, 83.7 million people will be older than 65 years by 2050.[3] The annual prevalence of chronic rhinosinusitis (CRS) is reported to be 13% to 16%.[4] The elderly represent a unique population to manage because of multiple medical comorbidities and polypharmacy.[5] The objective of this article is to discuss the diagnosis, treatment, and surgical options related to rhinitis and sinusitis for the geriatric population.

RHINITIS

Rhinitis refers to a heterogeneous group of nasal disorders characterized by symptoms of sneezing, nasal itching, rhinorrhea, and nasal congestion.[6] As per **Box 1**, rhinitis is divided into 2 major categories: allergic rhinitis (AR) and nonallergic rhinitis

Disclosure: The authors have nothing to disclose.
Department of Head and Neck Surgery, UCLA, 200 UCLA Medical Plaza, Suite 550, Los Angeles, CA 90095, USA
* Corresponding author.
E-mail address: jeffsuh@mednet.ucla.edu

Otolaryngol Clin N Am 51 (2018) 803–813
https://doi.org/10.1016/j.otc.2018.03.008
0030-6665/18/© 2018 Elsevier Inc. All rights reserved.

Box 1
Types of rhinitis

Allergic rhinitis

Nonallergic rhinitis types
    Drug induced
    Hormonal
    Infectious/systemic
    Nonallergic rhinitis with eosinophilia syndrome
    Vasomotor/nonallergic rhinopathy

(NAR), which is differentiated into additional variants. In the elderly, AR and NAR can coexist.[7] As there are no current guidelines specific for the geriatric population, the overall management of rhinitis is similar to that of the general adult population.

ALLERGIC RHINITIS

According to the Clinical Practice Guideline by the American Academy of Otolaryngology Head and Neck Surgery (AAO-HNS), AR is defined as a symptomatic nasal disorder mediated by immunoglobulin E (IgE)-mediated immune responses.[8] Allergens in the environment are taken up upon inhalation and deposited into the nasal mucosa. Subsequent inflammatory responses lead to an immediate allergic response and a late phase T-cell response.[9] Allergens include perennial allergens (dust mites, cockroach, pets) and seasonal allergens (grasses, trees, ragweeds). Coinciding with symptoms, physical findings on anterior rhinoscopy may show abundant clear mucus and enlarged turbinates with pale or boggy mucosa.

Diagnosis of Allergic Rhinitis

In addition to history and physical examination, current guidelines strongly recommend allergy testing for the diagnosis of AR.[8] Testing provides knowledge into the offending allergen, the total serum and specific IgE concentrations, and a target for immunotherapy. Although older adults have lower total IgE levels compared with younger patients, atopic disease is still present.[10]

Medical Treatment of Allergic Rhinitis

Similar to the general adult population, treatment of AR in the elderly includes environmental control, pharmacotherapy, immunotherapy, and potentially, surgery. For medical therapy, the AAO-HNS strongly recommends intranasal glucocorticosteroids and second-generation oral antihistamine drugs as first-line therapies.[8] Intranasal antihistamines are an option, especially in combination with intranasal steroids. Oral leukotriene receptor antagonists are not recommended as primary treatment.

    The AAO-HNS guidelines do not discuss decongestants, nasal irrigations, intranasal anticholinergics, or cromolyn sodium for the treatment of rhinitis. However, the Allergic Rhinitis and its Impact on Asthma (ARIA) guidelines do examine these medications, but not as first-line therapy.[11] Intranasal decongestants may be used for a short duration in patients with severe nasal obstruction. Oral decongestants may be indicated for symptom relief, but is strongly advised against in patients with cardiac conditions. Nasal irrigation with isotonic sodium chloride is indicated in patients with nasal dryness.[12] Topical chromones are modestly effective and safe. Topical anticholinergics are effective in controlling watery rhinorrhea, but not effective with sneezing or nasal obstruction. Further descriptions of these medications can be examined in **Table 1**.

Table 1
Pharmacotherapy for allergic rhinitis

Medication	Mechanism of Action	Side Effect	AAO-HNS Guideline	ARIA Guideline	Additional Comments
Intranasal steroids	Potently reduce nasal inflammation Reduce nasal hyperreactivity	Minor local side effects (burning, epistaxis)	Strongly recommend	Most effective pharmacologic	Maximal effect after a few days with daily compliance
Oral antihistamines	Blockage of H_1 receptor	First generation: sedation is common with anticholinergic effect Second generation: fewer side effects, limited by renal and liver function	Strongly recommend second generation	Second-generation oral antihistamines preferred	Effective in combination with intranasal steroids; rapidly effective (<1 h) on nasal and ocular symptoms
Nasal antihistamines	Blockage of H_1 receptor Some anti-allergic	Minor local side effects; bitter taste	Option, especially in combination with intranasal steroids	Effective	Rapidly effective (<30 min) on nasal or ocular symptoms
Leukotriene antagonists	Block CystLT receptor	Excellent tolerance	Recommend against as primary option	Effective on rhinitis and asthma, but inferior to intranasal steroids	

(continued on next page)

Table 1
(continued)

Medication	Mechanism of Action	Side Effect	AAO-HNS Guideline	ARIA Guideline	Additional Comments
Intranasal anticholinergic	Blocks almost exclusively rhinorrhea	Minor local side effects Almost no systemic anticholinergic activity	Not addressed	Effective on rhinorrhea	Does not affect sneezing or nasal obstruction
Intranasal chromones	Mast cell stabilization	Minor local side effects	Not addressed	Modestly effective	Intranasal chromones are less effective and the effect is short lasting
Oral decongestants	Sympathomimetic effect	Hypertension Palpitations Restlessness Agitation Tremor Insomnia Headache Dry mucous membranes Urinary retention Exacerbation of glaucoma or thyrotoxicosis	Not addressed	Use oral decongestants with caution in patients with heart disease; do not regularly use	Oral H1-antihistamine–decongestant combination products may be more effective than either product alone but side effects are combined
Intranasal decongestants	Sympathomimetic effect	Same as oral decongestant, but to less degree; rhinitis medicamentosa	Not addressed	Act more rapidly and more effectively than oral decongestants; do not regularly use	Limit duration of treatment to <3 d to avoid rhinitis medicamentosa

Pharmacotherapy of Allergic Rhinitis in the Geriatric Population

The literature shows no specific differences in the pharmacotherapy of AR for the geriatric population. However, the main concern is interactions between medications or between medications and comorbidities. Bozek[7] examines differences in pharmacotherapy of AR in the geriatric population. For intranasal steroids, no studies suggest increased side effects. Antileukotrienes, intranasal antihistamines, and intranasal anticholingerics are generally well tolerated.

Bozek[7] further describes the potential adverse effects of antihistamines, mainly first-generation types, and decongestants and advises caution with their use. Oral decongestant drugs may cause arterial hypertension, headache, and aggravation of glaucoma. First-generation antihistamines can cause several adverse effects: confusion, sedation, arrhythmias, and coordination problems. Second-generation antihistamines, although generally safer, should be cautiously used in patients with liver or kidney impairment.

Immunotherapy for Allergic Rhinitis in the Geriatric Population

According to the AAO-HNS guidelines, immunotherapy is strongly recommended for patients with AR who have persistent symptoms despite maximal pharmacologic therapy.[8] Immunotherapy allows for allergy desensitization and is given subcutaneously with shots or sublingually with drops. Maintenance of therapy requires regular intervals up to 3 to 5 years.[13]

Few studies have shown the efficacy and safety of immunotherapy in the geriatric population.[14,15] Immunotherapy does have its limitations in the elderly. For example, patients who regularly take β-blockers or ACE inhibitors are at higher risk of anaphylaxis.[16] Prolonged therapy makes it difficult for compliance in the elderly.[7]

Surgery for Allergic Rhinitis

The AAO-HNS recommends inferior turbinate reduction surgery in AR patients with nasal airway obstruction and enlarged inferior turbinates who have failed medical management.[8] There are no specific data on inferior turbinate reduction outcomes in geriatric patients. There are several different methods of turbinate reduction: turbinate out fracture, radiofrequency reduction, submucosal resection, and partial/complete resection. There are many different considerations that might lead a surgeon to choose one technique over another. However, the literature supports submucosal turbinate resection as having the longest efficacy.[17] For geriatric patients unable to tolerate general anesthesia, radiofrequency ablation can be done safely with good results in the office under local anesthesia.

NONALLERGIC RHINITIS

NAR is characterized by intermittent or persistent symptoms of nasal symptoms that are not due to an IgE-inflammatory response. As shown in **Box 1**, there are various forms of NAR that make diagnosis difficult based on symptoms alone. Two forms of NAR in the elderly are vasomotor rhinitis (VMR) and medication-induced rhinitis.

VASOMOTOR RHINITIS/NONALLERGIC RHINOPATHY

VMR/nonallergic rhinopathy is a form of NAR that is an idiopathic variant, generally thought to be caused by autonomic nervous system dysfunction.[18] The hallmark symptom is clear watery rhinorrhea, less often with congestion and sneezing. Potential triggers include temperature changes, gustatory stimuli, strong odors, passive tobacco smoke, and emotional factors.

The proposed pathophysiology is thought to be caused by autonomic dysfunction.[19] For example, rhinorrhea is a common symptom of patients with Parkinson disease.[20] VMR is a diagnosis of exclusion and is generally thought to be more prevalent in the elderly. However, there are few data suggesting clinical differences in the geriatric population. VMR responds particularly well to intranasal ipratropium bromide, which is generally considered to be safe.[19] However, narrow-angle glaucoma is a relative contraindication to the use of ipratropium.[21]

In terms of surgical options, vidian neurectomy may be offered as a last resort to patients with persistent, disabling symptoms refractory to medical therapy. The surgery's goal is disruption of the nasal cavity's autonomic supply to reduce nasal secretions.[22] Although studies have shown the safety and efficacy of vidian neurectomy,[23] there are no specific data in the geriatric population.

MEDICATION-INDUCED RHINITIS

Rhinitis can be caused by use of oral and topical medications (**Table 2**), which is important in the setting of polypharmacy. *Rhinitis medicamentosa* results from an overuse of topical α-adrenergic decongestant sprays. Chronic use causes rapid intolerance and severe rebound nasal congestion. Patients present with rhinorrhea, chronic sniffling, and sometimes debilitating nasal obstruction. Treatment is based on identification of the offending medication and substitution, if possible, with nasal irrigation and steroid sprays. For rhinitis medicamentosa, no data specifically studied the geriatric population.

OTHER CAUSES OF NONALLERGIC RHINITIS

Systemic diseases may present with symptoms of rhinitis and must be in the differential for NAR. Rheumatologic diseases, such as Wegener granulomatosis and sarcoidosis, are common considerations and require specific testing and treatment. Infectious rhinitis, most commonly, is due to a viral infection from rhinovirus. Other microbial causes include tuberculosis, rhinoscleroma, and fungus. Hormone imbalance, such as in menopause, can lead to rhinitis.[24] Last, malignancies may present with symptoms of rhinitis and should be investigated with nasal endoscopy and potentially imaging modalities. Unilateral symptoms or symptoms refractory to medical therapy should be further evaluated.

Table 2
Medications that can cause nonallergic rhinitis

Oral Medications	Topical Nasal Sprays/Drugs
Acetylsalicylic acid/nonsteroidal anti-inflammatory drugs	Oxymetazoline/Afrin
α-Blockers	Ephedrine
ACE inhibitors	Phenylephrine/Neo-Synephrine
β-Blockers	Amphetamines
Calcium channel blockers	Cocaine
Diuretics	
Phosphodiesterase 5 inhibitors	
Psychotropics	

SINUSITIS IN THE GERIATRIC POPULATION

The International Consensus Statement on Allergy and Rhinology (ICAR) and European Position Paper on Rhinosinusitis and Nasal Polyps (EPOS) provide clinical guidelines for acute sinusitis and chronic sinusitis for the adult population.[25,26] The management of sinusitis in the geriatric population will be similar to that of adults, with special consideration for potential drug interactions and side effects and medical comorbidities.

Managing CRS in the geriatric population can have a significant impact on QOL and should not be neglected. The health care costs of CRS[27] and the effects on QOL are well studied in the general adult population. Although these studies do not specifically focus on the elderly, the effect of CRS on QOL does have significant implications in the geriatric population. For example, depression has been linked with worse QOL metrics and with increased reliance on health care usage.[28]

ACUTE RHINOSINUSITIS

Per ICAR and EPOS, acute rhinosinusitis (ARS) is defined as sudden onset of 2 or more of the symptoms of nasal obstruction, purulent nasal drainage, reduction or loss of smell, and facial pain/pressure for less than 12 weeks.[25,26] Acute viral rhinosinusitis is usually characterized by mild symptoms less than 10 days; it is usually self-limiting without the need for prescription medications.

Acute bacterial rhinosinusitis (ABRS) is described as symptoms lasting beyond 10 days with unilateral pain, fever, elevated ESR/CRP, and deterioration after an initial milder phase. The most common bacteria are *Streptococcus pneumoniae*, *Haemophilus influenzae*, and *Moraxella catarrhalis*.[29] *Staphylococcus aureus* and *Streptococcus pyogenes* have a higher propensity to cause intracranial or orbital complications.[30]

Management of Acute Rhinosinusitis

Medical therapy is the mainstay for ARS. According to guidelines, initial therapy is nasal saline irrigation, analgesics, and topical nasal steroids. Antihistamines and systemic steroids are strongly not recommended. In ABRS, antibiotic therapy is recommended. Amoxicillin is considered first-line therapy.[29] For patients with penicillin allergy, trimethoprim-sulfamethoxazole or macrolide antibiotics can be used. Special consideration should be taken for medical therapy in the geriatric population. Antibiotic side effects (gastrointestinal upset, dizziness, and fatigue) may be increased in the elderly.[31] Radiologic imaging is generally not recommended unless an alternative diagnosis is suspected, the illness is severe, or concern for orbital or intracranial sequelae is present.[29]

CHRONIC RHINOSINUSITIS
Definition and Diagnosis

According to guidelines, CRS is defined by symptoms (nasal obstruction, nasal drainage, facial pain/pressure, and decreased sense of smell) for greater than 12 weeks.[25,26] Evaluation with nasal endoscopy or computed tomographic imaging is required in the current guidelines. Findings such as mucopurulence, nasal polyposis, or mucosal edema on endoscopy, or sinus opacification on imaging differentiate the symptoms from rhinitis or other conditions.

CRS is divided into CRS without nasal polyps (CRSsNP) versus CRS with polyps (CRSwNP). Patients with CRSwNP may require additional specialized care and long-term treatment to prevent polyp regrowth. Screening for allergic symptoms should be performed because allergy management plays an important role. Polyps, specifically unilateral disease, can be indistinguishable from neoplasms or encephaloceles, which should be in the differential diagnosis.[32]

Aging Impact on Pathogenesis of Chronic Rhinosinusitis

The pathogenesis of CRS consists of a complex inflammatory and infectious process. Microbial imbalance in the sinonasal mucosa may play a role in disease persistence.[33] Limited studies in the geriatric population have shown increased proportions of *S aureus* with decreased levels of *Corynebacterium* and *Propionibacterium*.[34] The data on the aging nasal microbiome are limited.

Mucociliary function is crucial in maintaining healthy sinuses, and thus, dysfunction is often a precursor to CRS.[35] In the geriatric population, there is decreased mucociliary clearance and thinning of nasal mucosa.[36] There is also a decrease in percent water per body weight in the elderly, leading to thicker mucus secretion.[37]

Aging effects on the immune system may predispose the elderly to CRS. For innate immunity, epithelial integrity is a key factor in impeding inhaled pathogens and allergens.[38] In the sinonasal tissue of patients older than 60 years old, studies have shown a decrease in the S100 protein, which mediates inflammatory activity, defends against pathogens, and promotes epithelial repair.[39,40]

The geriatric population may have difficulty mounting adaptive immune responses because of *immunosenescence,* which is age-related changes that contribute to increased susceptibility to infections, malignancy, and autoimmunity.[41] Chronic and subclinical systemic inflammation associated with aging in the absence of infection has been described.[42]

In summary, most studies on CRS in the geriatric population show potential differences in the pathogenesis of sinusitis. Further research is required for examining the clinical impact of these differences in CRS in the geriatric population.

Management of Chronic Rhinosinusitis

According to guidelines, medical therapy is the mainstay for the initial management of CRSsNP and CRSwNP.[25,26] Topical corticosteroid sprays and saline irrigation are the 2 key and proven therapies. Intranasal steroids do carry a risk of epistaxis, which is a common complaint of geriatric patients and especially important in those who are taking blood thinners.[43]

Antimicrobials are not recommended for the treatment of CRS, unless there are symptoms related to an exacerbation. Longer courses of culture-directed antibiotics are generally recommended to treat acute exacerbations (>2 weeks). According to EPOS, there is some evidence of long-term antibiotic therapy (>12 weeks) benefit with low-dose macrolides in CRSsNP with normal IgE levels.[26] Topical and intravenous antibiotics are not generally recommended for patients with CRS, but can be useful in select cases.

Systemic corticosteroids for short-term management are primarily reserved for severe exacerbations of CRS.[44] The side-effect profile of oral steroids includes insomnia, acid reflux, and mood changes and is relatively contraindicated in patients with osteoporosis, diabetes, glaucoma, and psychiatric illness, which are prevalent in the elderly population.

Surgical Management of Chronic Rhinosinusitis

Endoscopic sinus surgery (ESS) is recommended for severe or recalcitrant CRS patients, especially those who have little to no improvement with medical therapy.[25,26] Studies have shown improvement in symptoms, QOL, and postoperative endoscopic examination findings.[45] In the geriatric population, ESS is safe and efficacious in patients older than 60 years old with improvement in QOL metrics.[46,47]

Contributing Comorbidities in Chronic Rhinosinusitis

Comorbidities play a role in CRS development. Reflux of gastric acid into the nasopharynx has been shown to cause inflammation of the sinus ostium.[48] Gastroesophageal reflux disease is common in the elderly and is a diagnostic challenge given the absence of symptoms or presence of atypical symptoms, such as cough or voice changes.[49]

Smoking is a significant risk factor for the development of CRS and more importantly persistence of disease despite therapy.[50] Mucociliary clearance is impaired in cigarette smoke exposure. Smokers older than 60 years old are less likely than younger smokers to attempt quitting, and the benefits of cessation are somewhat less among the elderly.[51]

SUMMARY

Rhinitis and sinusitis are common medical conditions that affect the geriatric population and have a significant impact on their QOL. Because few studies examine differences in the clinical management between the geriatric and general adult population, therapies should be based on current guidelines as outlined by the AAO-HNS, EPOS, and ICAR. Special considerations should be made when treating these patients in regards to multiple comorbidities and the potential for drug interactions from polypharmacy. Further research on the pathogenesis of sinusitis in the geriatric population may provide specific differences in the clinical management in this population.

REFERENCES

1. DeConde AS, Soler ZM. Chronic rhinosinusitis: epidemiology and burden of disease. Am J Rhinol Allergy 2016;30(2):134–9.
2. Campbell AP, Phillips KM, Hoehle LP, et al. Depression symptoms and lost productivity in chronic rhinosinusitis. Ann Allergy Asthma Immunol 2017;118(3): 286–9.
3. Ortman JM, Velkoff VA, Hogan H. An aging nation: the older population in the United States. 2014. Available at: https://www.census.gov/content/dam/Census/library/publications/2014/demo/p25-1140.pdf. Accessed May 30, 2017.
4. Benninger MS, Ferguson BJ, Hadley JA, et al. Adult chronic rhinosinusitis: definitions, diagnosis, epidemiology, and pathophysiology. Otolaryngol Head Neck Surg 2003;129(3 suppl):S1–32.
5. Antimisiaris D, Cutler T. Managing polypharmacy in the 15-minute office visit. Prim Care 2017;44(3):413–28.
6. Wallace DV, Dykewicz MS, Bernstein DI, et al. The diagnosis and management of rhinitis: an updated practice parameter. J Allergy Clin Immunol 2008;122(2): S1–84.
7. Bozek A. Pharmacological management of allergic rhinitis in the elderly. Drugs Aging 2017;34(1):21–8.
8. Seidman MD, Gurgel RK, Lin SY, et al. Clinical practice guideline: allergic rhinitis. Otolaryngol Head Neck Surg 2015;152(1 suppl):S1–43.
9. Dykewicz MS, Hamilos DL. Rhinitis and sinusitis. J Allergy Clin Immunol 2010; 125(2 Suppl 2):S103–15.
10. Nyenhuis S, Mathur S. Rhinitis in older adults. Curr Allergy Asthma Rep 2013; 13(2):171–7.

11. Bousquet J, Khaltaev N, Cruz AA, et al. Allergic rhinitis and its impact on asthma (ARIA) 2008. Allergy 2008;63:8–160.
12. Yilmaz Sahin AA, Corey JP. Rhinitis in the elderly. Curr Allergy Asthma Rep 2006; 6:125–31.
13. Ozdemir C, Kucuksezer UC, Akdis M, et al. Mechanisms of aeroallergen immunotherapy. Immunol Allergy Clin North Am 2016;36(1):71–86.
14. Bozek A, Ignasiak B, Filipowska B, et al. House dust mite sublingual immunotherapy: a double-blind, placebo-controlled study in elderly patients with allergic rhinitis. Clin Exp Allergy 2012;43:242–8.
15. Asero R. Efficacy of injection immunotherapy with ragweed and birch pollen in elderly patients. Int Arch Allergy Immunol 2004;135:332–5.
16. Jutel M, Agache I, Bonini S, et al. International consensus on allergen immunotherapy II: mechanisms, standardization, and pharmacoeconomics. J Allergy Clin Immunol 2016;137(2):358–68.
17. Bhandarkar ND, Smith TL. Outcomes of surgery for inferior turbinate hypertrophy. Curr Opin Otolaryngol Head Neck Surg 2010;18(1):49–53.
18. Jaradeh SS, Smith TL, Torrico L, et al. Autonomic nervous system evaluation of patients with vasomotor rhinitis. Laryngoscope 2000;100:1828–31.
19. Loehrl TA. Autonomic dysfunction, allergy and upper airway. Curr Opin Otolaryngol Head Neck Surg 2007;15(4):264–7.
20. Chou KL, Koeppe RA, Bohnen NI. Rhinorrhea: a common nondopaminergic feature of Parkinson's disease. Mov Disord 2011;26(2):320–3.
21. Ah-kee EY, Egong E, Shafi A, et al. A review of drug-induced acute angle closure glaucoma for non-ophthalmologists. Qatar Med J 2015;2015(1):6.
22. Robinson SR, Wormald PJ. Endoscopic vidian neurectomy. Am J Rhinol 2006;20: 197–202.
23. Marshak T, Yun WK, Hazout C, et al. A systematic review of the evidence base for vidian neurectomy in managing rhinitis. J Laryngol Otol 2016;130(Suppl 4): S7–28.
24. Choi JH, Hwang SH, Suh JD, et al. Menopausal hormone therapy may increase non-allergic rhinitis among postmenopausal women: results from the Korea National Health and Nutrition Examination Survey (2010–2012). Maturitas 2017; 102:46–9.
25. Orlandi RR, Kingdom TT, Hwang PH. International consensus statement on allergy and rhinology: rhinosinusitis executive summary. Int Forum Allergy Rhinol 2016;6:S3–21.
26. Fokkens WJ, Lund VJ, Mullol J, et al. European position paper on rhinosinusitis and nasal polyps 2012. Rhinol Suppl 2012;23:1–298.
27. Murphy MP, Fishman P, Short SO, et al. Health care utilization and cost among adults with chronic rhinosinusitis enrolled in a health maintenance organization. Otolaryngol Head Neck Surg 2002;127(5):367–76.
28. Schlosser RJ, Gage SE, Kohli P, et al. Burden of illness: a systematic review of depression in chronic rhinosinusitis. Am J Rhinol Allergy 2016;30(2):250–6.
29. Rosenfeld RM, Andes D, Bhattacharyya N, et al. Clinical practice guideline: adult sinusitis. Otolaryngol Head Neck Surg 2007;137(suppl):S1–31.
30. Meltzer EO, Hamilos DL, Hadley JA, et al. Rhinosinusitis: establishing definitions for clinical research and patient care. Otolaryngol Head Neck Surg 2004;131(6): S1–62.
31. Rosenfeld RM, Singer M, Jones S. Systematic review of antimicrobial therapy in patients with acute rhinosinusitis. Otolaryngol Head Neck Surg 2007;137:S32–45.

32. London NR Jr, Reh DD. Differential diagnosis of chronic rhinosinusitis with nasal polyps. Adv Otorhinolaryngol 2016;79:1–12.
33. Stevens WW, Lee RJ, Schleimer RP, et al. Chronic rhinosinusitis pathogenesis. J Allergy Clin Immunol 2015;136:1442–53.
34. Ramakrishnan VR, Feazel LM, Gitomer SA, et al. The microbiome of the middle meatus in healthy adults. PLoS One 2013;8(12):e85507.
35. Hamilos DL. Host-microbial interactions in patients with chronic rhinosinusitis. J Allergy Clin Immunol 2014;133:640–53.
36. Ho JC, Chan KN, Hu WH, et al. The effect of aging on nasal mucociliary clearance, beat frequency, and ultrastructure of respiratory cilia. Am J Respir Crit Care Med 2001;163:983–8.
37. DelGaudio JM, Panella NJ. Presbynasalis. Int Forum Allergy Rhinol 2016;6: 1083–7.
38. Tieu DD, Kern RC, Schleimer RP. Alterations in epithelial barrier function and host defense responses in chronic rhinosinusitis. J Allergy Clin Immunol 2009;124: 37–42.
39. Tieu DD, Peters AT, Carter RT, et al. Evidence for diminished levels of epithelial psoriasin and calprotectin in chronic rhinosinusitis. J Allergy Clin Immunol 2010;125:667–75.
40. Cho SH, Hong SJ, Han B, et al. Age-related differences in the pathogenesis of chronic rhinosinusitis. J Allergy Clin Immunol 2012;129:858–60.
41. Shaw AC, Goldstein DR, Montgomery RR. Age-dependent dysregulation of innate immunity. Nat Rev Immunol 2013;13:875–87.
42. Franceschi C, Campisi J. Chronic inflammation (inflammaging) and its potential contribution to age-associated diseases. J Gerontol 2014;69(suppl 1):S4–9.
43. Özler GS, Yengil E. Why do geriatric patients visit otorhinolaryngology? Ear Nose Throat J 2016;96(6):224–9.
44. Smith KA, Rudmik L. Medical therapy, refractory chronic rhinosinusitis, and productivity costs. Curr Opin Allergy Clin Immunol 2017;17(1):5–11.
45. Smith TL, Litvack JR, Hwang PH, et al. Determinants of outcomes of sinus surgery: a multi-institutional prospective cohort study. Otolaryngol Head Neck Surg 2010;142(1):55–63.
46. Colclasure JC, Gross CW, Kountakis SE. Endoscopic sinus surgery in patients older than sixty. Otolaryngol Head Neck Surg 2004;131(6):946–9.
47. Jiang RS, Hsu CY. Endoscopic sinus surgery for the treatment of chronic sinusitis in geriatric patients. Ear Nose Throat J 2001;80(4):230–2.
48. Schreiber S, Garten D, Sudhoff H. Pathophysiological mechanisms of extraesophageal reflux in otolaryngeal disorders. Eur Arch Otorhinolaryngol 2009;266: 17–24.
49. Soumekh A, Schnoll-Sussman FH, Katz PO. Reflux and acid peptic diseases in the elderly. Clin Geriatr Med 2014;30(1):29–41.
50. Briggs RD, Wright ST, Cordes S. Smoking in chronic rhinosinusitis: a predictor of poor long-term outcome after endoscopic sinus surgery. Laryngoscope 2009; 119(11):2269–74.
51. Burn DM. Cigarette smoking among the elderly: disease consequences and the benefits of cessation. Am J Health Promot 2000;14(6):357–61.

Age-Related Deficits in Taste and Smell

Richard L. Doty, PhD

KEYWORDS

- Olfaction • Gustation • Taste • Smell • Age • Geriatrics • Psychophysics

KEY POINTS

- Taste and smell decline markedly with age, greatly impacting safety, food intake, and quality of life.
- In the case of smell, more than one-half of the population between 65 and 80 years have demonstrable loss; over 80 years this increases to more than three quarters.
- Environmental factors play a significant role in producing age-related smell loss and likely swamp genetic factors later in life. Smell loss in older populations significantly impacts the likelihood of mortality over the course of 4 to 5 years.
- Reasons for age-related smell loss include cumulative damage to the olfactory receptor cells, ossification of the foramina of the cribriform plate, and changes in neural responsiveness.
- Several age-related neurodegenerative diseases exhibit smell loss, most notably Alzheimer's and Parkinson's diseases. Such loss occurs, in many cases, decades before the classic diagnostic phenotype.

INTRODUCTION

The ability to taste and smell significantly declines later in life.[1,2] This phenomenon is perhaps best illustrated for the sense of smell; more than one-half of those between the ages of 65 and 80 years, and more than 75% of those over the age of 80 years, have a demonstrable decline.[3] Such dysfunction impacts quality of life, including the flavor of foods and beverages, as well as safety. In a study of 750 consecutive patients presenting to the University of Pennsylvania Smell and Taste Center for evaluation, 68% reported a decreased quality of life, 46% a change in appetite or body weight, and 56% a negative impact on daily living or psychological well-being.[4] A study of more than 1000 patients conducted at the Medical College of Virginia found

Disclosure: The author receives funding from the Michael J. Fox Foundation for Parkinson's Research. He is a consultant to Acorda Therapeutics, Eisai Co, Ltd, and Johnson & Johnson. He receives royalties from Cambridge University Press, Johns Hopkins University Press, and John Wiley & Sons, Inc. He is President of, and a major shareholder in, Sensonics International, a manufacturer and distributor of smell and taste tests.

Smell and Taste Center, Department of Otorhinolaryngology, Head and Neck Surgery, Perelman School of Medicine, University of Pennsylvania, Philadelphia, PA 19104, USA
E-mail address: doty@mail.med.upenn.edu

Otolaryngol Clin N Am 51 (2018) 815–825
https://doi.org/10.1016/j.otc.2018.03.014
0030-6665/18/© 2018 Elsevier Inc. All rights reserved.

that those who could not smell (anosmics) were 3 times more likely than normosmics to have experienced a potentially life-threatening event at some point in their lives, including ingestion of spoiled food or the failure to detect smoke or leaking natural gas.[5] Remarkably, healthy older anosmics are also 3 times more likely to die over a subsequent 4- to 5-year period than their normosmic peers, although the cause of this difference is unknown.[6,7] The same risk also occurs in acutely hospitalized older patients with significant taste loss.[8]

This review describes the basic anatomy and physiology of the senses of smell and taste and discusses the functional and pathophysiologic changes that occur in these senses in the later years of life. The goal is to provide the clinician with a fundamental understanding of these changes and information for evaluating, treating, and counseling older patients with chemosensory disturbances.

BASIC ANATOMY OF THE TASTE AND SMELL SYSTEMS
The Taste System

Tastants are sensed by specialized microvillus receptor cells found in approximately 8000 taste buds located throughout the oral cavity. Most taste buds, which also contain supporting and basal cells from which the other cells are derived (**Fig. 1**),[9] are embedded within the fungiform, foliate, and circumvallate papillae of the tongue.

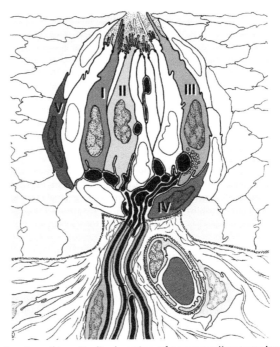

Fig. 1. Idealized drawing of longitudinal section of a mammalian taste bud. Cells of types I, II, and III are elongated. These cells have different types of microvilli within the taste pit and may reach the taste pore. Type IV are basal cells and type V are marginal cells. Classically defined synapses occur only between type III cells and nerve fibers. Many of the connecting taste nerves have myelin sheaths. (*From* Witt M, Reutter K. Anatomy of the tongue and taste buds. In: Doty RL, editor. Handbook of Olfaction and Gustation. 3rd edition. Hoboken (NJ): John Wiley & Sons; 2015. p. 638; with permission.)

Others are found within the mucosa of the uvula, soft palate, rostral esophagus, and laryngeal surface of the epiglottis. Sweet and umami (savory) taste sensations are mediated via G-protein-coupled receptor proteins located on receptor cell microvilli within the buds. Three genes (TAS1R1-TAS1R3) encode sweet receptors, whereas at least 60 genes encode bitter receptors (TAS2R1-TAST2R60). Salty taste, for example that produced by sodium chloride, requires the diffusion of the Na^+ ions through specialized membrane channels, such as the amiloride-sensitive Na^+ channel. Sour tastes are likely mediated via the PKD2L1 receptor, a member of the transient receptor potential protein family.[10]

The taste buds are innervated by 3 cranial nerves (cranial nerves VII, IX and X). Cranial nerve VII supplies the buds of the anterior tongue, as well as those of the palate. Cranial nerve IX supplies those on the foliate and circumvallate papillae, whereas cranial nerve X supplies those in the larynx and esophagus.[11] The nucleus tractus solitarius of the brainstem receives projections from the afferent nerves that synapse with taste bud receptor cells. These axons synapse in an orderly rostral to caudal fashion within the nucleus tractus solitarius—those from cranial nerve VII synapse rostral to those from cranial nerve IX, which in turn synapse rostral to those from cranial nerve X. Projections from the nucleus tractus solitarius go to the thalamus and, from there, to the primary taste cortex at the junction of the anterior insula and the inner operculum. Subsequent projections occur to other cortical regions where multisensory interactions take place.[12]

It is important to note that many so-called taste receptors are found outside the oral cavity, most notably in the alimentary and respiratory tracts. For example, α-gustducin, the taste-specific G-protein α-subunit, is expressed in brush cells within the human trachea, lung, pancreas, and gallbladder. These cells are rich in nitric oxide synthase and aid in mucosal defense against xenobiotic organisms and acid-induced lesions. Some T2R bitter receptors are expressed in the motile cilia of the human airway. They play a role in increasing ciliary beat frequency when stimulated with bacteria-related compounds, including acyl-monoserine lactone quorum-sensing molecules secreted by *Pseudomonas aeruginosa* and other gram-negative bacteria.[13] Interestingly, persons who are tasters of the bitter tasting agent phenylthiocarbamide express more of these cells than nontasters and are less susceptible to nasal sinus disease.[14]

The Olfactory System

Volatiles enter the highest recesses of the nose from either the external nares (orthonasal) or from the oral cavity via the nasopharynx (retronasal) and dissolve in the mucus that overlies the olfactory epithelium.[15,16] This pseudostratified squamous epithelium lines the cribriform plate and superior sectors of the nasal septum, middle turbinate, and superior turbinate. Once dissolved, odorants bind to receptors on the olfactory receptor cells.[15] When damaged, olfactory receptor cells can be replaced by stem cells located near the basement membrane, although this process is often incomplete. Thus, the adult olfactory epithelium is typically pot-marked with islands of invading respiratory epithelium.

Bundles of axons of the ciliated olfactory receptor cells (termed fila) coalesce within the lamina propria of each side of the nose and subsequently project through the cribriform plate to the ipsilateral olfactory bulb, an outgrowth of the forebrain (**Fig. 2**).[17] Within the olfactory bulb, the olfactory receptor cell axons synapse with second order neurons, most notably the mitral and tufted cells. Considerable modulation of the incoming information occurs in the bulb (for a review, see Doty 2015[18]). The mitral and tufted cell axons project via the lateral olfactory tract to multiple regions of the ipsilateral temporal lobe.

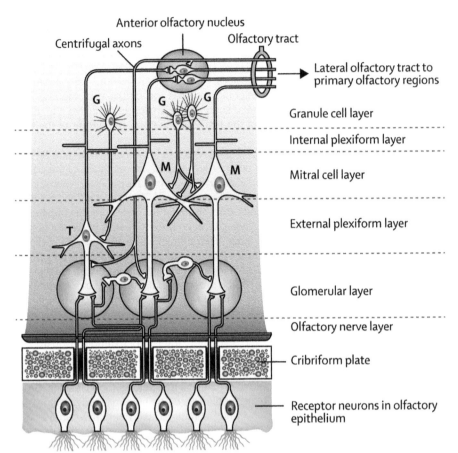

Fig. 2. Diagram of the main cell types and layers of the olfactory bulb, the first relay station of the olfactory system. The bulb is located at the base of the brain immediately over the cribriform plate and receives axons from the olfactory receptor cells. These axons synapse with dendrites of the main output neurons, the mitral and tufted cells, within glomeruli, which are spherical masses of neuropile that make up a distinct layer of the bulb. Cells located between the glomeruli (periglomerular cells) often extend across several glomeruli. Note the centrifugal input from central brain regions onto the granule (G), mitral (M), and tufted (T) cells. (*From* Duda JE. Olfactory system pathology as a model of Lewy neurodegenerative disease. J Neurol Sci 2010;289(1–2):50; with permission.)

Like taste receptors, olfactory receptors have been identified outside the olfactory epithelium, including in the bladder, blood vessels, heart, intestine, kidney, skin, skeletal muscle, lungs, pancreas, prostate, testes, thyroid, thymus, and ganglia of the autonomic nervous system.[19] As with the case of ectopic taste receptors, they are likely misnamed and should be viewed as generalized chemoreceptors whose function depends on where in the body they are expressed.

AGE-RELATED CHANGES IN TASTE AND SMELL PERCEPTION
Taste

The influence of age on taste function is well-established. However, considerable variability exists and such declines do not occur in all persons. An example of the

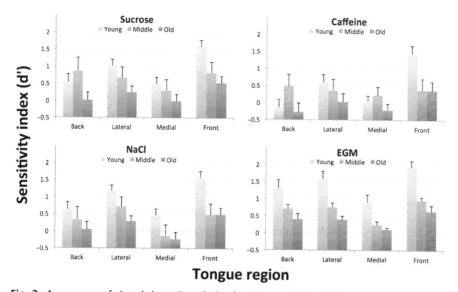

Fig. 3. A measure of signal detection–derived taste sensitivity (d') for 3 age groups and 4 tongue regions for sucrose, caffeine, and sodium chloride, and electric current (electrogustometry; EGM). Note the age-related decrement in performance for all measures, as well as differences between tongue regions. (*From* Doty RL, Heidt JM, MacGillivray MR, et al. Influences of age, tongue region, and chorda tympani nerve sectioning on signal detection measures of lingual taste sensitivity. Physiol Behav 2016;155:205; with permission.)

average age-related declines in sensitivity of small regions of the tongue to chemical and electrical taste stimuli is shown in **Fig. 3**.[20] In this study, dry filter paper disks previously soaked in tastants were applied to different regions of the tongue, and an electrogustometer—a device that produces low electrical currents (**Fig. 4**)—was

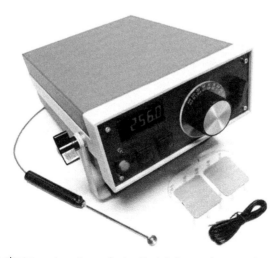

Fig. 4. A modern electrogustometer, a device that delivers microamp-level currents to a disk electrode placed on the tongue. (*Courtesy of* Sensonics International. Copyright © 2017 Sensonics International, Haddon Heights, NJ.)

used to present the electrical stimuli. Electrogustometry requires no rinsing between stimulus presentations and taste buds can be easily stimulated at remote locations (eg, deep in the oral cavity and on the soft palate). However, the classic taste qualities are not reliably induced, even though, as seen in **Fig. 3**, electrical responses largely mirror those obtained from chemical tastants for different regions of the tongue and for different age groups.

Olfaction

Age-related decrements in the ability to smell are evident for all types of olfactory tests, including nominal tests of odor identification, detection, discrimination, and memory. In cognitively intact older adults, olfactory loss can be predictive, to some degree, of future cognitive decline, as well as to the transition from mild cognitive impairment to Alzheimer's disease.[21,22]

An example of the decline in the ability to identify odors is presented in **Fig. 5**, as measured by the University of Pennsylvania Smell Identification Test (**Fig. 6**). In this test, 40 odorants are presented on scratch and sniff labels and the subject is required to choose the correct odor from a list of 4 alternatives, that is, the test is forced choice. This format allows for the detection of malingering on the basis of avoiding the correct responses at too high a rate.

It is important to emphasize that most complaints of "taste" loss reflect altered olfactory function. Thus, sensations that are commonly viewed as taste (eg, coffee, chocolate, pizza, apple, strawberry) are mediated through the olfactory system. During deglutition, these tastes result from retronasal stimulation of the olfactory receptors via the nasal pharynx.[23] Because the intensity of mastication and swallowing can be less in some older persons as a result of slower and weaker mouth movements, the amount air that is forced through the nasopharynx is decreased, thereby mitigating the taste experience. The term flavor is preferred for describing the whole taste experience related to not only olfaction and taste, but to oral somatosensation as well.

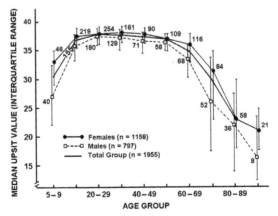

Fig. 5. Scores on the University of Pennsylvania Smell Identification Test (UPSIT; see **Fig. 6**) as a function of subject age and sex. Numbers by each datapoint indicate sample sizes. Note that women identify odorants better than men at all ages. (*From* Doty RL, Shaman P, Applebaum SL, et al. Smell identification ability: changes with age. Science 1984;226(4681):1442; with permission.)

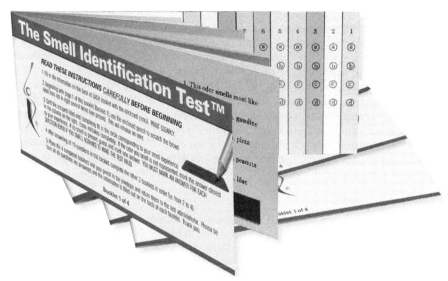

Fig. 6. The University of Pennsylvania Smell Identification Test (UPSIT), known commercially as the Smell Identification Test. (*Courtesy of* Sensonics International. Copyright © 2017 Sensonics International, Haddon Heights, NJ.)

THE PHYSIOLOGIC BASIS FOR AGE-RELATED CHEMOSENSORY ALTERATIONS
The Oral Taste System

The cause of the changes in taste with age are multiple. Salient among the causes are malnutrition, diabetes, and xerostomia.[24] Neurologic and oral epithelial changes are also evident. Thus, declines in taste bud numbers with age is prevalent in some tongue regions.[25] For example, Arey and colleagues[25] found that the mean number of buds per circumvallate papilla to be 248 in 43 individuals ranging from less than 1 to 20 years of age, 206 in 38 individuals 20 to 70 years of age, and 88 in 13 individuals 74 to 85 years of age. However, histologic studies of taste buds in fungiform papillae of rodents, monkeys, and humans do not show meaningful age-related declines.[26–28]

Relatively little is known about age-related changes in the central nervous system that impact taste function. Green and colleagues[29] found that, during hedonic evaluation of sweet (sucrose) and bitter (caffeine) tasting stimuli, greater bilateral activation on functional MRI in young than middle-aged adults within sensory (insula) and reward (lentiform nucleus) regions for sucrose, but not for caffeine. The young adults had greater responses during hedonic evaluation of sucrose than of caffeine in several sensory and motor processing regions (precentral and postcentral gyri, insula), but there were no taste-related differences in activation in the middle-aged adults. These findings suggested the possibility that middle age decrements in taste function may be precursors of decrements that occur in the elderly.

A number of taste distortions (dysgeusias) or hallucinations (phantogeusias) seem to be induced by medications, particularly in the elderly, where polypharmacy is a significant problem. Nearly three-quarters of antihyperlipidemic drugs listed in the *Physician's Desk Reference* are associated with taste complaints, including such common drugs as atorvastatin calcium (Lipitor), fluvastatin (Lescol), pravastatin (Provachol), and lovastatin (Mevacor), and simvastatin (Zocor). More.than one-third of antihypertensive drugs reportedly have adverse taste side effects, including calcium channel blockers, diuretics (eg, amiloride), and angiotensin-converting enzyme inhibitors. Among angiotensin-converting enzyme inhibitors, captopril is particularly problematic, being associated with complaints of ageusia and a range of taste distortions (metallic, bitter, salty).[30,31] The basis of such drug-related taste problems is poorly understood, although alterations of ion channels is likely in some cases.[32]

It is rarely appreciated that poor dental hygiene can impact taste function in the elderly. One study found, for example, that elderly persons who received professional oral hygiene therapy 3 times a week for 5 weeks exhibited a lowering of thresholds for sucrose and sodium chloride relative to controls, who were similarly visited by an oral hygienist who only inspected and swabbed their teeth.[33] Additionally, poorly fitting dentures can impact mastication and the general taste of foods in addition to retronasal flavor perception.

The Olfactory System

There are several causes for age-related decline in olfactory function, some of which may also be applicable to the declines observed in taste function. First, exposures to air pollution, cigarette smoke, viruses, bacteria, and other airborne xenobiotics cumulatively damage the olfactory epithelium, as noted. Such exposures have more functional consequence in later years when the cumulative effects become more manifest.[34–36] Second, age is associated with retarded receptor cell regeneration. In the rat, the ratio of live receptor cells to dead or dying cells decreases with aging.[37] Repair of the olfactory epithelium is slower or nonexistent in older mice whose epithelium has been chemically damaged.[38,39] Third, an age-related decrease in the size and number of patent foramina of the cribriform plate results in blocking the passage of olfactory receptor cell axons into the brain from the nasal cavity and induces necrosis in many olfactory receptor cells.[40,41] Fourth, immunologic and enzymatic defense mechanisms critical for maintaining the integrity of the epithelium decrease in older age. These mechanisms include expression of phase I and phase II xenobiotic metabolizing enzymes, such as epithelial carnosinase, glutathione, S-transferases, heat-shock protein 70, and isoforms of cytochrome P-450.[42–44] Fifth, age compromises the response specificity of individual olfactory receptor cells. For example, biopsied receptor cells from older persons exhibit broader electrophysiologic tuning curves than do such receptor cells from younger persons.[45] Sixth, neuropathology associated with such age-related diseases as Alzheimer's and Parkinson's diseases invade olfactory eloquent brain regions in later life, seeming to impact function.[46]

The role genes play in influencing age-related changes in olfactory function is not clear. Older persons homozygous for the val allele of the val66met polymorphism of brain-derived neurotrohic factor experience a greater 5-year decrease in odor identification performance than older persons heterozygous for this allele (v/m) or homozygous for the met allele (m/m).[47] Older carriers of the ε4-allele of the human apolipoprotein E gene, a plasma protein involved in lipid transport, similarly exhibit more longitudinal declines in odor identification than noncarriers.[48] This decrease occurs even after controlling for the effects of vocabulary and general cognitive status, suggesting that the influences of this allele on odor perception are largely independent of clinical dementia.[49] Twin studies suggest that environmental factors likely swamp age-related genetic factors in determining the degree of olfactory function in the elderly.[50]

SUMMARY

Disturbances in the ability to smell and to taste are common in older persons. Such disturbances can significantly influence nutrition, safety, and quality of life, as well as both psychological and physical health. The anatomic and physiologic causes of age-related disturbances are multiple and interacting, and depend on genetic and environmental factors. Frank losses of function, as well as distortions and hallucinations, are common. Fortunately, most distortions resolve over time, although this can, in some instances, can take months or even years.[51] It is now known that olfactory dysfunction occurs during the very earliest stages of a number of neurologic disorders, most notably Alzheimer's disease and Parkinson's disease, likely heralding the onset of the underlying disease process.

REFERENCES

1. Doty RL, Kamath V. The influences of age on olfaction: a review. Front Psychol 2014;5:20.
2. Methven L, Allen VJ, Withers CA, et al. Ageing and taste. Proc Nutr Soc 2012; 71(4):556–65.
3. Doty RL, Shaman P, Applebaum SL, et al. Smell identification ability: changes with age. Science 1984;226:1441–3.
4. Deems DA, Doty RL, Settle RG, et al. Smell and taste disorders, a study of 750 patients from the University of Pennsylvania Smell and Taste Center. Arch Otolaryngol Head Neck Surg 1991;117:519–28.
5. Pence TS, Reiter ER, DiNardo LJ, et al. Risk factors for hazardous events in olfactory-impaired patients. JAMA Otolaryngol Head Neck Surg 2014;140: 951–5.
6. Pinto JM, Wroblewski KE, Kern DW, et al. Olfactory dysfunction predicts 5-year mortality in older adults. PLoS One 2014;9:e107541.
7. Devanand DP, Lee S, Manly J, et al. Olfactory identification deficits and increased mortality in the community. Ann Neurol 2015;78:401–11.
8. Solemdal K, Moinichen-Berstad C, Mowe M, et al. Impaired taste and increased mortality in acutely hospitalized older people. Chem Senses 2014;39:263–9.
9. Witt M, Reutter K. Anatomy of the tongue and taste buds. In: Doty RL, editor. Handbook of olfaction and gustation. 3rd edition. Hoboken (NJ): John Wiley & Sons; 2015. p. 637–64.
10. Roper SD. Signal transduction and information processing in mammalian taste buds. Pflugers Arch 2007;454:759–76.
11. Witt M, Reutter K. Anatomy of the tongue and taste buds. In: Doty RL, editor. Handbook of olfaction and gustation. 3rd edition. New York: Wiley-Liss; 2015. p. 639–65.
12. Pritchard TC, Di Lorenzo PM. Central taste anatomy and physiology of rodents and primates. In: Doty RL, editor. Handbook of olfaction and gustation. Hoboken (NJ): John Wiley & Sons; 2015. p. 701–26.
13. Lee RJ, Xiong G, Kofonow JM, et al. T2R38 taste receptor polymorphisms underlie susceptibility to upper respiratory infection. J Clin Invest 2012;122:4145–59.
14. Adappa ND, Howland TJ, Palmer JN, et al. Genetics of the taste receptor T2R38 correlates with chronic rhinosinusitis necessitating surgical intervention. Int Forum Allergy Rhinol 2013;3:184–7.
15. Ding X, Xie F. Olfactory mucosa: composition, enzymatic localization, and metabolism. In: Doty RL, editor. Handbook of olfaction and gustation. 3rd edition. Hoboken (NJ): John Wiley & Sons; 2015. p. 63–92.
16. Yoshikawa K, Touhara K. Olfactory receptor function. In: Doty RL, editor. Handbook of olfaction and gustation. 3rd edition. Hoboken (NJ): John Wiley & Sons; 2015. p. 109–21.

17. Ennis M, Holy TE. Anatomy and neurobiology of the main and accessory olfactory bulbs. In: Doty RL, editor. Handbook of olfaction and gustation. 3rd edition. Hoboken (NJ): John Wiley & Sons; 2015. p. 157–82.

18. Doty RL, editor. Handbook of olfaction and gustation. 3rd edition. Hoboken (NJ): John Wiley & Sons; 2015. p. 1–1217.

19. Ferrer I, Garcia-Esparcia P, Carmona M, et al. Olfactory receptors in non-chemosensory organs: the nervous system in health and disease. Front Aging Neurosci 2016;8:163.

20. Doty RL, Heidt JM, MacGillivray MR, et al. Influences of age, tongue region, and chorda tympani nerve sectioning on signal detection measures of lingual taste sensitivity. Physiol Behav 2016;155:202–7.

21. Conti MZ, Vicini-Chilovi B, Riva M, et al. Odor identification deficit predicts clinical conversion from mild cognitive impairment to dementia due to Alzheimer's disease. Arch Clin Neuropsychol 2013;28:391–9.

22. Devanand DP, Tabert MH, Cuasay K, et al. Olfactory identification deficits and MCI in a multi-ethnic elderly community sample. Neurobiol Aging 2010;31:1593–600.

23. Burdach KJ, Doty RL. The effects of mouth movements, swallowing, and spitting on retronasal odor perception. Physiol Behav 1987;41:353–6.

24. Bromley SM, Doty RL. Clinical disorders affecting taste: an update. In: Doty RL, editor. Handbook of olfaction and gustation. 3rd edition. Hoboken (NJ): John Wiley & Sons; 2015. p. 887–910.

25. Arey LB, Tremaine MJ, Monzingo FL. The numerical and topographical relations of taste buds to human circumvallate papillae throughout the life span. Anat Rec 1935;64:9–25.

26. Arvidson K. Location and variation in number of taste buds in human fungiform papillae. Scand J Dent Res 1979;87:435–42.

27. Bradley RM, Stedman HM, Mistretta CM. Age does not affect numbers of taste buds and papillae in adult rhesus monkeys. Anat Rec 1985;212:246–9.

28. Miller IJ Jr. Human taste bud density across adult age groups. J Gerontol 1988; 43:B26–30.

29. Green E, Jacobson A, Haase L, et al. Can age-related CNS taste differences be detected as early as middle age? Evidence from fMRI. Neuroscience 2013;232: 194–203.

30. Grosskopf I, Rabinovitz M, Garty M, et al. Persistent captopril-associated taste alteration. Clin Pharm 1984;3:235.

31. McNeill JJ, Anderson A, Christophidis N, et al. Taste loss associated with oral captopril treatment. Br Med J 1979;2:1555–6.

32. Zervakis J, Graham BG, Schiffman SS. Taste effects of lingual application of cardiovascular medications. Physiol Behav 2000;68:405–13.

33. Langan MJ, Yearick ES. The effects of improved oral hygiene on taste perception and nutrition of the elderly. J Gerontol 1976;31:413–8.

34. Loo AT, Youngentob SL, Kent PF, et al. The aging olfactory epithelium: neurogenesis, response to damage, and odorant-induced activity. Int J Dev Neurosci 1996; 14:881–900.

35. Hirai T, Kojima S, Shimada A, et al. Age-related changes in the olfactory system of dogs. Neuropathol Appl Neurobiol 1996;22:531–9.

36. Smith CG. Age incidence of atrophy of olfactory nerves in man. J Comp Neurol 1942;77:589–94.

37. Mackay-Sim A, St John J, Schwob JE. Neurogenesis in the adult olfactory epithelium. In: Doty RL, editor. Handbook of olfaction and gustation. 3rd edition. Hoboken (NJ): John Wiley & Sons; 2015. p. 133–56.

38. Matulionis DH. Effects of the aging process on olfactory neuron plasticity. In: Breipohl W, editor. Olfaction and endocrine regulation. London: IRL Press; 1982. p. 299–308.
39. Breipohl W, Mackay-Sim A, Grandt D, et al. Neurogenesis in the vertebrate main olfactory epithelium. In: Breipohl W, editor. Ontogeny of olfaction. Berlin: Springer-Verlag; 1986. p. 21–33.
40. Kalmey JK, Thewissen JG, Dluzen DE. Age-related size reduction of foramina in the cribriform plate. Anat Rec 1998;251:326–9.
41. Krmpotic-Nemanic J. Presbycusis, presbystasis and presbyosmia as consequences of the analogous biological process. Acta Otolaryngol 1969;67:217–23.
42. Krishna NS, Getchell TV, Dhooper N, et al. Age- and gender-related trends in the expression of glutathione S-transferases in human nasal mucosa. Ann Otol Rhinol Laryngol 1995;104:812–22.
43. Kirstein CL, Coopersmith R, Bridges RJ, et al. Glutathione levels in olfactory and non-olfactory neural structures of rats. Brain Res 1991;543:341–6.
44. Getchell TV, Krishna NS, Dhooper N, et al. Human olfactory receptor neurons express heat shock protein 70: age-related trends. Ann Otol Rhinol Laryngol 1995; 104:47–56.
45. Rawson NE, Gomez G, Cowart B, et al. The use of olfactory receptor neurons ORNs. from biopsies to study changes in aging and neurodegenerative diseases. Ann N Y Acad Sci 1998;855:701–7.
46. Braak H, de VR, Jansen EN, et al. Neuropathological hallmarks of Alzheimer's and Parkinson's diseases. Prog Brain Res 1998;117:267–85.
47. Hedner M, Nilsson LG, Olofsson JK, et al. Age-related olfactory decline is associated with the BDNF Val66met polymorphism: evidence from a population-based study. Front Aging Neurosci 2010;2:24.
48. Calhoun-Haney R, Murphy C. Apolipoprotein epsilon4 is associated with more rapid decline in odor identification than in odor threshold or Dementia Rating Scale scores. Brain Cogn 2005;58:178–82.
49. Olofsson JK, Nordin S, Wiens S, et al. Odor identification impairment in carriers of ApoE-varepsilon4 is independent of clinical dementia. Neurobiol Aging 2010;31: 567–77.
50. Doty RL, Petersen I, Mensah N, et al. Genetic and environmental influences on odor identification ability in the very old. Psychol Aging 2011;26:864–71.
51. Deems DA, Yen DM, Kreshak A, et al. Spontaneous resolution of dysgeusia. Arch Otolaryngol Head Neck Surg 1996;122:961–3.

Sleep Apnea and Sleep-Disordered Breathing

Jiahui Lin, MD[a], Maria Suurna, MD[b],*

KEYWORDS

- Obstructive sleep apnea • Snoring • Elderly • Geriatric • Sleep-disordered breathing
- CPAP

KEY POINTS

- Changes in sleep rhythm, duration, and architecture are normal aspects of aging; it is important to distinguish these changes from symptoms of an underlying sleep disorder.
- The prevalence of undiagnosed sleep apnea and sleep-disordered breathing is high in the elderly.
- These disorders may have a significant impact on quality of life as well as increase associated mortality and morbidity, if left untreated.
- Initial treatment of obstructive sleep apnea is positive airway pressure, which has been shown to improve quality of life as well as morbidity and mortality.

INTRODUCTION

Sleep apnea and sleep-disordered breathing are prevalent disorders in the adult population and are often associated with a wide variety of comorbid conditions. Most common disorders that fall under the category of sleep-disordered breathing include obstructive sleep apnea (OSA), central sleep apnea, and sleep-related hypoventilation. Degree of airway narrowing can range from snoring to complete collapse of the airway with cessation of airflow. As the rate of obesity, particularly in Western societies, has been steadily increasing, associated higher prevalence of sleep-disordered breathing has been also observed. In-laboratory polysomnography is considered the gold standard for diagnosis of clinically suspected sleep-related breathing disorders in adults. A home sleep test is an alternative diagnostic method for patients with no major comorbid conditions, although it carries some limitations. Diagnosis of sleep apnea is established in the presence of respiratory events resulting

Disclosure: Dr M. Suurna, MD is an investigator in clinical trial for Inspire Medical.
[a] Department of Otolaryngology–Head and Neck Surgery, New York-Presbyterian Hospital, Columbia and Weill Cornell, 180 Fort Washington Avenue, New York, NY 10032, USA; [b] Department of Otolaryngology–Head and Neck Surgery, Weill Cornell Medicine, New York Presbyterian Hospital, 1305 York Avenue, New York, NY 10021, USA
* Corresponding author.
E-mail address: mas9390@med.cornell.edu

0030-6665/18/© 2018 Elsevier Inc. All rights reserved.

in an apnea-hypopnea index (AHI) of at least 5 events per hour in symptomatic patients. This article focuses on the impact of these disorders and management strategies in the older adult patients.

EPIDEMIOLOGY OF SLEEP DISORDERS IN THE ELDERLY

A survey from the National Sleep Foundation showed that among adults between 55 and 84 years of age, 52% reported a sleep problem. The described sleep-associated problems included difficulty falling asleep, frequent awakenings, early awakening, awakening unrefreshed, daytime sleepiness, pauses in breathing, snoring, unpleasant feeling in the legs, or less than 6 hours of nightly sleep.[1] Population-based studies have shown that symptomatic OSA affects approximately 3% to 7% of adult men and 2% to 5% of adult women.[2] Other studies have shown that the prevalence of OSA, both symptomatic and asymptomatic, is 20% and 56% in women, and 28% and 70% in men between the ages of 65 and 99 years defined by AHI and respiratory disturbance index (RDI) of at least 10 events per hour, respectively.[3] Other population-based studies showed that in adults older than 65, the prevalence of OSA is as high as 90% in men and 78% in women.[4,5] However, most age-related increases in the prevalence of OSA occur before the age of 65 years.[6] Indeed, the Sleep Heart Health Study found that the increase in prevalence of OSA appeared to plateau after the age of 65 years.[7] Nevertheless, these studies highlight a significant proportion of undiagnosed and occult sleep-disordered breathing in the aging population.

PATHOPHYSIOLOGY

Collapse of the pharyngeal and retrolingual airway is the primary cause of obstruction in OSA. Many factors may contribute to this collapse. The genioglossus is considered to be most important muscle in maintaining airway patency. Studies have shown that older adults have a decreased genioglossus response and lower neuromuscular tone, which may contribute to their increased rate of OSA.[8] Menopause is another risk factor for sleep-disordered breathing, likely related to estrogen depletion.[6,9] Interestingly, survey data show that changes in body mass index (BMI) are only weakly associated with changes in AHI, and the association between AHI and obesity is even weaker in older adults.[7,10] Furthermore, snoring and symptoms of daytime sleepiness are reported less frequently among older adults despite the increase in OSA prevalence.[6] Explanations for these findings could be the fact that bed partners who typically report on snoring are no longer alive or, because of age-related factors, do not hear the snoring. Older adults also are more likely to have components of central apnea. Regardless of the cause, sleep-disordered breathing is a more complex entity in older adults and should be recognized through detailed history taking and physical examination.

CHANGING SLEEP PATTERNS IN THE ELDERLY

Sleep patterns change as adults age (**Box 1**).[11] Changes such as sleep rhythm, duration, and architecture in older adults have been well documented. A survey from the National Sleep Foundation showed that 33% of older adults reported fair or poor quality of sleep, and 13% reported having a diagnosis of a sleep disorder.[1] Oftentimes, older adults have various comorbid conditions that interfere with sleep, including depression, prostate hypertrophy, gastroesophageal reflux, arthritis, and pulmonary disorders (**Box 2**). Many medications can also cause nocturia, such as diuretics, and are taken commonly in this patient population. On average, total sleep time decreases by 10 minutes per decade of life.[12,13] Sleep onset latency also increases

> **Box 1**
> **Changes in sleep patterns in the elderly**
>
> - Fewer continuous hours asleep at night
> - Increased daytime naps
> - Increased sleep latency
> - Decreased sleep efficiency
> - Decreased REM sleep
> - Increased sleep fragmentation

with age. Moreover, slow-wave sleep and rapid eye movement (REM) sleep also decrease in the elderly.

Despite the many changes in sleep patterns, most older adults are able to maintain normal alertness during the day. Thus, when older adults present with excessive daytime sleepiness, this should alert the clinician that other factors may be at play, such as sleep-disordered breathing. However, normal age-related changes may be difficult to differentiate from changes from an underlying sleep disorder, the most common of which are OSA and restless leg syndrome in this population.[14] Obtaining a detailed sleep history, as well as any comorbid conditions that could be contributing, may help in the diagnosis. Furthermore, polypharmacy is common in the elderly, and many medications may contribute to sleep disturbances. Eliciting history of caffeine, nicotine, and alcohol use is also important. Helping patients understand the effect of these substances on sleep as well as medication adjustments and management of co-morbid disorders may improve sleep quality.

COMPLICATIONS OF SLEEP-DISORDERED BREATHING IN THE ELDERLY

Sleep disorders are widely known to be associated with comorbidities, such as hypertension and cardiac disease. In a survey from the National Sleep Foundation, 40% of older adults with major comorbidities, such as hypertension, arthritis, heart disease, diabetes, depression, cancer, lung disease, osteoporosis, memory problems, stroke, and enlarged prostate, reported that their sleep quality was fair or poor. In contrast, only 10% without these conditions reported fair or poor quality of sleep.[1]

> **Box 2**
> **Causes of sleep disturbance in the elderly**
>
> - Natural changes in sleep patterns with age (see **Box 1**)
> - Sleep-disordered breathing and sleep apnea
> - Restless leg syndrome
> - Depression
> - Prostate hypertrophy
> - Gastroesophageal reflux
> - Arthritis
> - Pulmonary disorders
> - Medications causing nocturia

Patients with sleep apnea and other sleep disorders often have decreased cognitive function. A meta-analysis of 13 studies showed a statistically significant impact on neuropsychological performance in older adults with OSA.[15] Processing speed and declarative memory were found to be affected in particular. OSA has been found to be significantly associated with decreased psychomotor efficiency in the Wisconsin Sleep Cohort Study.[16] Sleep-disordered breathing in the elderly has been found to negatively impact cognition, including attention, executive function, and memory.[17] It has been postulated that age may exert a synergistic effect with sleep-disordered breathing to affect cognitive decline, although more studies are needed to elucidate this relationship. Other studies have shown similar effects of OSA on cognitive function.[10,18]

Sleep-disordered breathing and OSA have been shown to negatively impact quality of life, including general health perception, physical functioning, social functioning, and vitality.[6] OSA has been shown to be associated with depression in elderly patients and thus leads to lower quality of life.[19] It has been shown that use of continuous positive airway pressure (CPAP) in patients with moderate to severe OSA can improve quality of life measures, such as reduction in sleepiness, anxiety, and depression.[20] Interestingly, other studies have found that sleep apnea has little to no significant impact on overall quality of life measures in the elderly.[21,22] However, the effects of aging on these quality measures are often difficult to separate out from the effects of sleep-disordered breathing.

The association between OSA and mortality has been well studied. Studies have shown an increase of associated cardiovascular mortality in elderly patients with OSA.[23] Furthermore, it has also been shown that in elderly the treatment of OSA with CPAP may decrease the risk of all-cause and cardiovascular mortality.[23–25] Even just having symptoms of OSA, such as snoring and excessive daytime sleepiness, is associated with an increased risk of heart failure in women.[26] Similarly, snoring has been shown to be associated with ischemic heart disease and stroke in men.[27]

Hypertension has been found to be increased in patients with OSA. Population-based studies have shown increasing blood pressure associated with increasing AHI.[28,29] Large population studies, including large numbers of adults older than the age of 65 years, have also shown linear associations increased AHI and blood pressure, even after adjusting for BMI.[30] Because of the increase in cardiovascular mortality in OSA patients with concomitant hypertension, it has been postulated that hypertension may be an important cause of cardiovascular mortality in OSA.[31] Studies have shown variable results in blood pressure reduction after initiation of CPAP therapy.[32] However, CPAP treatment may have some benefit in decreasing blood pressure in patients with more severe OSA and more severe hypertension.[33] Management of cardiovascular risk factors with strong adherence to CPAP therapy has broader overall health benefits, rather than individual effects on a particular comorbidity.

Other associated health risks have been well studied in OSA. Peripheral arterial occlusive disease has been associated with OSA and sleep-disordered breathing, but this association becomes insignificant after adjusting for confounding variables, such as hypertension, hyperlipidemia, and diabetes.[34,35] Such results do not discount the detrimental risks of OSA; rather, they point to the fact that the contribution of OSA to these latter variables may thus indirectly increase risks for yet other comorbidities.

TREATMENT

Management of OSA often requires a multidisciplinary approach. The initial treatment of choice for OSA is positive airway pressure (PAP), which can be delivered as CPAP, bilevel PAP, or autotitrating PAP. Studies have shown improvement in not only day-time sleepiness but also morbidity and mortality with the use of CPAP in the elderly.[23,24,33,36] Behavioral treatment options should be addressed with the patient. The treatment may include weight loss, positional therapy, and avoidance of alcohol and sedatives before bedtime. Oral appliances can be used as an adjunct or alternative to CPAP therapy options. A mandibular advancement device has been shown to improve OSA symptoms, although CPAP generally provided more benefit.[36,37]

Various surgical treatment options are available for the management of OSA and sleep-disordered breathing. Because of higher associated morbidity, surgical treatment is usually considered for patients for whom PAP therapy and oral appliances do not provide adequate treatment. Therapy is usually directed at the site of obstruction and is often staged.[38] Nasal surgeries include septoplasty, inferior turbinate reduction, adenoidectomy, and nasal valve reconstruction. Procedures for palatal obstruction include tonsillectomy and uvulopalatopharyngoplasty and its modifications. Hypopharyngeal surgeries include lingual tonsillectomy, partial midline glossectomy, mandibular osteotomy, genioglossal advancement, hyoid myotomy and suspension, as well as maxillomandibular osteotomy and advancement. Newer technologies such as hypoglossal nerve stimulation implant are becoming more appealing as alternatives to the CPAP treatment option because of lower associated surgical morbidity, good clinical outcomes, and the multilevel effect on airway obstruction.[39,40] However, surgical treatments of OSA and sleep-disordered breathing in the elderly are not well studied, in part because of the higher prevalence of comorbid conditions and increased risks associated with general anesthesia in this patient population. In healthy, older individuals with significant sleep-disordered breathing or OSA with CPAP intolerance, individualized surgical treatment options should be considered.

SUMMARY

Older adults undergo gradual changes in their sleep patterns, and it is important to differentiate normal age-related sleep changes from sleep disorders. As sleep disorders can impact an older adult's day-to-day life and contribute to various comorbidities, these patients should be carefully screened with a detailed medical history, combined with a detailed sleep history. There is evidence to support a high prevalence of undiagnosed sleep apnea in the elderly. Timely diagnosis and treatment of sleep-disordered breathing not only may provide benefit to quality of life but may also improve associated morbidity and mortality.

REFERENCES

1. Foley D, Ancoli-Israel S, Britz P, et al. Sleep disturbances and chronic disease in older adults: results of the 2003 National Sleep Foundation Sleep in America Survey. J Psychosom Res 2004;56:497–502.
2. Punjabi NM. The epidemiology of adult obstructive sleep apnea. Proc Am Thorac Soc 2008;5:136–43.
3. Ancoli-Israel S, Kripke DF, Klauber MR, et al. Sleep-disordered breathing in community-dwelling elderly. Sleep 1991;14:486–95.
4. Senaratna CV, Perret JL, Lodge CJ, et al. Prevalence of obstructive sleep apnea in the general population: a systematic review. Sleep Med Rev 2017;34:70–81.
5. Heinzer R, Vat S, Marques-Vidal P, et al. Prevalence of sleep-disordered breathing in the general population: the HypnoLaus study. Lancet Respir Med 2015;3: 310–8.

6. Young T, Peppard PE, Gottlieb DJ. Epidemiology of obstructive sleep apnea: a population health perspective. Am J Respir Crit Care Med 2002;165:1217–39.

7. Young T, Shahar E, Nieto FJ, et al. Predictors of sleep-disordered breathing in community-dwelling adults: the Sleep Heart Health Study. Arch Intern Med 2002;162:893–900.

8. Klawe JJ, Tafil-Klawe M. Age-related response of the genioglossus muscle EMG-activity to hypoxia in humans. J Physiol Pharmacol 2003;54(Suppl 1):14–9.

9. Young T, Finn L, Austin D, et al. Menopausal status and sleep-disordered breathing in the Wisconsin Sleep Cohort Study. Am J Respir Crit Care Med 2003;167: 1181–5.

10. Ancoli-Israel S, Gehrman P, Kripke DF, et al. Long-term follow-up of sleep disordered breathing in older adults. Sleep Med 2001;2:511–6.

11. Piani A, Brotini S, Dolso P, et al. Sleep disturbances in elderly: a subjective evaluation over 65. Arch Gerontol Geriatr Suppl 2004;(9):325–31.

12. Ohayon MM, Carskadon MA, Guilleminault C, et al. Meta-analysis of quantitative sleep parameters from childhood to old age in healthy individuals: developing normative sleep values across the human lifespan. Sleep 2004;27:1255–73.

13. Zalai D, Bingeliene A, Shapiro C. Sleepiness in the elderly. Sleep Med Clin 2017; 12:429–41.

14. Barthlen GM. Sleep disorders. Obstructive sleep apnea syndrome, restless legs syndrome, and insomnia in geriatric patients. Geriatrics 2002;57:34–9 [quiz: 40].

15. Cross N, Lampit A, Pye J, et al. Is obstructive sleep apnoea related to neuropsychological function in healthy older adults? A systematic review and meta-analysis. Neuropsychol Rev 2017;27(4):389–402.

16. Kim HC, Young T, Matthews CG, et al. Sleep-disordered breathing and neuropsychological deficits. A population-based study. Am J Respir Crit Care Med 1997; 156:1813–9.

17. Zimmerman ME, Aloia MS. Sleep-disordered breathing and cognition in older adults. Curr Neurol Neurosci Rep 2012;12:537–46.

18. Adams N, Strauss M, Schluchter M, et al. Relation of measures of sleep-disordered breathing to neuropsychological functioning. Am J Respir Crit Care Med 2001;163:1626–31.

19. Farajzadeh M, Hosseini M, Mohtashami J, et al. The association between obstructive sleep apnea and depression in older adults. Nurs Midwifery Stud 2016;5:e32585.

20. McEvoy RD, Antic NA, Heeley E, et al. CPAP for prevention of cardiovascular events in obstructive sleep apnea. N Engl J Med 2016;375:919–31.

21. Appleton SL, Vakulin A, McEvoy RD, et al. Undiagnosed obstructive sleep apnea is independently associated with reductions in quality of life in middle-aged, but not elderly men of a population cohort. Sleep Breath 2015;19:1309–16.

22. Martinez-Garcia MA, Soler-Cataluna JJ, Roman-Sanchez P, et al. Obstructive sleep apnea has little impact on quality of life in the elderly. Sleep Med 2009; 10:104–11.

23. Martinez-Garcia MA, Campos-Rodriguez F, Catalan-Serra P, et al. Cardiovascular mortality in obstructive sleep apnea in the elderly: role of long-term continuous positive airway pressure treatment: a prospective observational study. Am J Respir Crit Care Med 2012;186:909–16.

24. Jennum P, Tonnesen P, Ibsen R, et al. Obstructive sleep apnea: effect of comorbidities and positive airway pressure on all-cause mortality. Sleep Med 2017;36: 62–6.

25. Nishihata Y, Takata Y, Usui Y, et al. Continuous positive airway pressure treatment improves cardiovascular outcomes in elderly patients with cardiovascular disease and obstructive sleep apnea. Heart Vessels 2015;30:61–9.
26. Ljunggren M, Byberg L, Theorell-Haglow J, et al. Increased risk of heart failure in women with symptoms of sleep-disordered breathing. Sleep Med 2016;17:32–7.
27. Koskenvuo M, Kaprio J, Telakivi T, et al. Snoring as a risk factor for ischaemic heart disease and stroke in men. Br Med J (Clin Res Ed) 1987;294:16–9.
28. Young T, Peppard P, Palta M, et al. Population-based study of sleep-disordered breathing as a risk factor for hypertension. Arch Intern Med 1997;157:1746–52.
29. Mokhlesi B, Finn LA, Hagen EW, et al. Obstructive sleep apnea during REM sleep and hypertension. Results of the Wisconsin Sleep Cohort. Am J Respir Crit Care Med 2014;190:1158–67.
30. Nieto FJ, Young TB, Lind BK, et al. Association of sleep-disordered breathing, sleep apnea, and hypertension in a large community-based study. Sleep Heart Health Study. JAMA 2000;283:1829–36.
31. Lavie P, Herer P, Peled R, et al. Mortality in sleep apnea patients: a multivariate analysis of risk factors. Sleep 1995;18:149–57.
32. Floras JS. Obstructive sleep apnea syndrome, continuous positive airway pressure and treatment of hypertension. Eur J Pharmacol 2015;763:28–37.
33. Kolanis S, Pilavakis M, Sofogianni A, et al. Is there a role for continuous positive airway pressure treatment in the management of obstructive sleep apnea-related hypertension? Curr Hypertens Rev 2017;13(2):89–92.
34. Chen JC, Koo M, Hwang JH. Risks of peripheral arterial occlusive disease in patients with obstructive sleep apnoea: a population-based case-control study. Clin Otolaryngol 2015;40:437–42.
35. Olson LG, King MT, Hensley MJ, et al. A community study of snoring and sleep-disordered breathing. Health outcomes. Am J Respir Crit Care Med 1995;152: 717–20.
36. Bratton DJ, Gaisl T, Schlatzer C, et al. Comparison of the effects of continuous positive airway pressure and mandibular advancement devices on sleepiness in patients with obstructive sleep apnoea: a network meta-analysis. Lancet Respir Med 2015;3:869–78.
37. Marklund M, Franklin KA. Treatment of elderly patients with snoring and obstructive sleep apnea using a mandibular advancement device. Sleep Breath 2015;19: 403–5.
38. Wakefield TL, Lam DJ, Ishman SL. Sleep apnea and sleep disorders. In: Flint PW, Haughey BH, Lund VJ, et al, editors. Cummings otolaryngology–head and neck surgery. Philadelphia: Elsevier; 2014. p. 252–70.
39. Sommer JU, Hormann K. Innovative surgery for obstructive sleep apnea: nerve stimulator. Adv Otorhinolaryngol 2017;80:116–24.
40. Strollo PJ, Soose RJ, Maurer JT, et al. Upper-airway stimulation for obstructive sleep apnea. N Engl J Med 2014;370(2):139–49.

Medical and Preoperative Evaluation of the Older Adult

Audrey Chun, MD

KEYWORDS

• Preoperative • Geriatric • Older adult • Surgery • Elderly • Function • Frailty

KEY POINTS

• Older adults have increased risks of postoperative complications because of physiologic changes and higher incidence of multiple chronic conditions.
• Comprehensive preoperative evaluation for older adults incorporates components of geriatric assessment, including evaluation of cognition, capacity, medication management, function, and frailty.
• Identified risks should be addressed with a problem-specific management plan to reduce risk.
• Surgical decisions should incorporate patient's preferences and expectations.

INTRODUCTION

Preoperative evaluation serves to identify potential risk and to optimize patients before surgery. Because of age, increased rates of multimorbidity, polypharmacy, functional changes, and cognitive impairment, older adults are at higher risk for perioperative complications. Identifying modifiable risk factors and educating patients and families about what to expect can improve surgical outcomes and satisfaction. Comprehensive preoperative evaluation assesses potential factors that may increase a patient's risk for complications. By 2030, more than 20% of Americans will be older than the age of 65 years and will account for a large number of planned and emergent procedures.[1] In response to these demographic changes, the American College of Surgeons National Surgical Quality Improvement Program (ACS NSQIP)/American Geriatrics Society (AGS) developed best practices guidelines that focus on the optimal preoperative assessment of the geriatric surgical patient. In contrast to the routine preoperative evaluation that concentrates on cardiac and pulmonary risk evaluation, the optimal preoperative evaluation for older adults addresses the following domains[2]:

1. Cognition/capacity, including memory and depression screens
2. Screening for alcohol and substance misuse

Disclosure: The author has nothing to disclose.
Department of Geriatrics and Palliative Medicine, Icahn School of Medicine at Mount Sinai, One Gustave Levy Place, Box 1070 New York, NY 10029, USA
E-mail address: audrey.chun@mssm.edu

Otolaryngol Clin N Am 51 (2018) 835–846
https://doi.org/10.1016/j.otc.2018.03.010
0030-6665/18/© 2018 Elsevier Inc. All rights reserved.

oto.theclinics.com

3. Delirium risk
4. Cardiac
5. Pulmonary
6. Function
7. Frailty
8. Nutrition
9. Medications
10. Patient counseling
11. Preoperative testing

DISCUSSION

Identification of cognitive impairment may affect the entire preoperative evaluation because of implications around capacity, decision-making, and also strongly predicting postoperative delirium, which is associated with worse surgical outcomes including longer length of stay, mortality and functional decline (**Box 1**).[3] For patients without known cognitive impairment, office-based screens, such as the Mini-Cog (three-item recall and clock draw) can quickly assess short-term memory, attention, and executive function.[4] Patients with identified cognitive impairment or known dementia should be counseled on their increased risk of postoperative delirium, its implications, and ways to mitigate risk.

Symptoms of cognitive impairment can sometimes be a manifestation of depression and depression screening should be included as part of cognitive assessment. Additionally, preoperative depression has been associated with increased mortality after certain cardiac procedures and also with higher pain perception and increased need for postoperative analgesic use.[2] Office screens can help identify patients who have depressive symptoms, and the Patient Health Questionnaire-2 is one screen consisting of two questions[5]: "In the past 12 months, have you ever had a time when you felt sad, blue, depressed, or down for most of the time for at least 2 weeks?"; and "In the past 12 months, have you ever had a time, lasting at least 2 weeks, when you didn't care about the things that you usually cared about or when you?"

Answering "yes" to either question suggests the need for additional evaluation and management for depression. Questions are asked by trained members of staff or through a written questionnaire.

All patients should also be evaluated for their capacity to consent to the procedure, especially if there is evidence of cognitive impairment. The patient should be able to demonstrate understanding of relevant information provided, acknowledgment of medical condition, treatment options and likely outcomes, clear indication of treatment choice, and engagement in rational discussion.[6] For those with evidence of cognitive impairment or diminished capacity, it is important to identify a surrogate

---

Box 1
Cognition/capacity

Assessment: Mini-Cog, Patient Health Questionnaire-2, capacity assessment

Action: educate on associated risks, establish health care proxy, document capacity

Data from Borson S, Scanlan J, Chen P, et al. The Mini-Cog as a screen for dementia: validation in a population-based sample. J Am Geriatr Soc 2003;51(10):1451–4; and Li C, Friedman B, Conwell Y, et al. Validity of the Patient Health Questionnaire 2 (PHQ-2) in identifying major depression in older people. J Am Geriatr Soc 2007;55:596–602.

Box 2
Alcohol/substance screening

Assessment: CAGE

Action: multivitamin with folate, thiamine; close monitoring for signs of withdrawal

Data from Hinkin C, Castellon S, Dickson-Fuhrman E, et al. Screening for drug and alcohol abuse among older adults using a modified version of the CAGE. Am J Addict 2001;10(4):319–26.

---

or proxy decision maker with whom the patient is comfortable and to establish if the procedure aligns with the patient's goals of care.

Preoperative alcohol misuse or abuse is associated with higher risk of mortality and complications including infections and longer length of stay (**Box 2**).[2] In addition to a cognitive assessment, the ACS NSQIP-AGS guidelines strongly recommend preoperative depression and substance abuse screening. A commonly used office screen for alcohol abuse is the CAGE questionnaire (Cut back, Annoyed, Guilt, Eye-opener), which has been validated in an older adult population.[7] Patients answering yes to any of these questions may indicate that the patient is at risk for alcohol misuse/abuse. Elective surgery should be delayed to allow time for treatment, if alcohol or substance abuse is verified. If surgery must proceed, the patient should begin a multivitamin with folate and thiamine, which should continue perioperatively, and the surgical team should be aware of the potential for withdrawal.

Delirium is the most common postoperative complication for older adults and potentially preventable in up to 40% of delirium cases (**Box 3**).[3] Delirium has been associated with increased rates of morbidity, mortality, functional loss, hospital costs, and length of stay.[8] Although some risk factors for delirium cannot be changed, others are potentially modifiable and should be optimized, if possible, before any procedure and continue perioperatively (**Box 4**).[2,3,8]

Based on the patient's individual risk factors, the intervention may include the following[3]:

- Discontinuation of unnecessary medications
- Cognitive reorientation before and after the procedure
- Mobility/functional support
- Adaptations for visual and hearing impairments
- Adequate hydration and nutrition
- Pain management
- Sleep enhancement (nonpharmacologic)
- Correction of any metabolic/electrolyte abnormalities
- Constipation management

Patients and families should be counseled on the possibility of delirium, its effects, and steps that they can take before and after the procedure to reduce the risks of developing postoperative delirium.

Box 3
Delirium risk

Assessment: assess risk factors

Action: implement management plan to mitigate modifiable risk factor, including education of patients and families

---

Box 4
Patient-related risk factors for delirium

- Older age greater than 70 y
- Cognitive impairment and dementia
- Severe illness or comorbidities
- Renal insufficiency

Potentially modifiable

- Anemia
- Hypoxia
- Electrolyte abnormalities
- Sleep deprivation
- Poor nutrition
- Dehydration
- Poor functional status
- Immobilization
- Hearing or vision impairment
- Polypharmacy and use of psychotropic medications
- Risk of urinary retention or constipation, presence of urinary catheter

---

Although cardiac complications occur in less than 4% of patients undergoing noncardiac surgery, even for those at high risk of cardiac disease, older adults are more vulnerable to complications of cardiac adverse events (**Box 5**).[9] Therefore, all patients should be evaluated for their perioperative cardiac risk according to the American College of Cardiology and American Heart Association algorithm for noncardiac surgery.[2,10]

Additionally, for patients on oral anticoagulation, there should be recommendations for if/when to stop, if bridging or reversal therapy is recommended, and when to resume oral therapy. This is determined by the indication for anticoagulation, type of anticoagulation medication, risk of thromboembolism off anticoagulation, risk of bleeding if anticoagulation is continued, and timing of surgery.[11,12] Reversal should occur for emergent surgery with high risk of bleeding, but generally is not needed for elective surgeries. For elective surgeries of average bleeding risk, timing of when to stop the anticoagulation agent is based on the effective half-life of the medication. Bridging therapy is generally not necessary except in situations where anticoagulation is indicated for the presence of a mechanical valve or a condition that places the patient at high risk of thromboembolic

---

Box 5
Cardiac

Assessment: American College of Cardiology and American Heart Association algorithm

Action: cardiac testing and optimization based on risk assessment

Data from Fleisher LA, Fleischmann KE, Auerbach AD, et al. 2014 ACC/AHA guideline on perioperative cardiovascular evaluation and management of patients undergoing noncardiac surgery: a report of the American College of Cardiology/American Heart Association Task Force on practice guidelines. J Am Coll Cardiol 2014;64(22):e77–137.

Box 6
Pulmonary

Assessment: history of pulmonary risk factors

Action: mitigate risk factors, as able; smoking cessation

---

events. Under most circumstances, anticoagulation can be resumed 24 to 72 hours after surgery, depending on the specific surgery and bleeding risk.

Postoperative pulmonary complications are common in patients with functional impairment or moderate to severe disease (American Society of Anesthesiologists class 3 or higher) (**Box 6**). These pulmonary complications are associated with increased early postoperative mortality, intensive care unit admission, and length of stay.[13] Preoperative evaluation should assess for pulmonary risk factors as follows[14,15]:

- Chronic lung disease, such as like asthma or chronic obstructive pulmonary disease (COPD)
- Obstructive sleep apnea
- Tobacco use
- Obesity
- Functional dependence
- Sensorium changes (vision/hearing loss)

Pending the time frame to surgery, strategies for preventing postoperative pulmonary complications include weight loss, smoking cessation, intensive respiratory muscle training, optimization of underlying lung disease (obstructive sleep apnea, COPD, and asthma symptom management), and selective pulmonary testing.[2,14]

Functional status assessment measures a person's ability to perform daily activities. It has great prognostic ability for perioperative outcomes, and impaired functional status has been associated with poor postoperative outcomes (**Box 7**).[16] A simple screening test to assess functional status consists of determining the patient's ability to get into and out of a chair unassisted, dress, bathe, toilet, feed, and groom (**Box 8**).[17]

If the patient/caregiver reports difficulty in performing any of these activities of daily living, a more in-depth screening needs to be performed and deficits documented. A history of falls or fear of falling should also be documented. Gait and mobility testing should be performed using the a standardized test, such as the Timed Up and Go Test, where a patient is asked to stand from a seated position, walk 15 feet, and return to the starting position and sit down.[18] Any patient requiring more than 15 seconds to complete the test is at high risk of falls. Prolonged Timed Up and Go Test, and any functional dependence, have been found to be strong predictors for institutional rehabilitation postoperatively.[2] Additionally, sensorineural deficits, such as vision or

---

Box 7
Function/falls

Assessment: Activities of daily living, hearing/vision screen, falls history, Timed Up and Go Test

Action: physical therapy, assistive support

Data from Katz S, Downs T, Cash H, et al. Progress in development of the index of AD. Gerontologist 1970;10:20–30; and Podsiadlo D, Richardson S. The timed "Up & Go": a test of basic functional mobility for frail elderly persons. J Am Geriatr Soc 1991;39:142–8.

Box 8
Katz index of activities of daily living-16

Bathing

Toileting

Dressing

Transferring

Continence

Feeding

---

hearing loss, should be documented with referrals for vision optimization and hearing amplifiers, as appropriate. Swallowing ability should also be noted, because this is important for postoperative nutrition.

Frailty has been identified as a predictor of surgical complications.[19,20] The syndrome of frailty refers to the decreased physiologic reserve that creates vulnerability to and difficulty in recovering from stressors (**Box 9**). Although several frailty measurement tools have been validated, most incorporate concepts related to sarcopenia, weakness, slow gait, low endurance, or energy. The Fried Frailty Index includes five items that address the phenotype of frailty and are assessed in a routine office visit: (1) unintentional weight loss greater than 10 lbs in the past year, (2) decreased grip strength, (3) self-reported poor energy and endurance, (4) low physical activity, and (5) slow walking.[19]

Each item receives a score of 0 (if not present) or 1 (if present), with a total score range of 0 to 5. Scores greater than two indicate frailty, and scores of one or two indicate prefrailty. Exercise prescriptions and "prehab" programs targeted at the phenotypic features of frailty may improve outcomes.[21,22]

For hospitalized surgical patients, malnutrition increases hospital length of stay and costs, and is associated with increased risk of adverse postoperative events (**Box 10**).[2,23] Assessment should include history of unintentional weight loss and documentation of baseline weight, height, and albumin. If available, and if time permits, patients identified to have poor nutrition benefit from referral to a dietician for a comprehensive nutritional plan to optimize nutritional status.[2] Nutrition recommendations may include modifications to diet, food consistency changes, and nutritional supplements. Compared with no intervention, dietary advice and/or nutritional supplements have been shown to improve weight, muscle bulk, and strength, although there is inconclusive evidence related to survival effects.[24] Patients with dentures should be reminded to bring them to the hospital to facilitate appropriate caloric intake postoperatively.[9]

Older adults are at risk of polypharmacy (more than five medications) because of increased incidence of multiple chronic conditions and often multiple specialty

---

Box 9
Frailty

Assessment: Fried Frailty Index

Action: exercise program, nutritional support, "prehab"

Data from Makary MA, Segev DL, Pronovost PJ, et al. Frailty as a predictor of surgical outcomes in older patients. J Am Coll Surg 2010;210(6):901–8.

Box 10
Nutrition

Assessment: serum albumin, body mass index, weight loss history

Action: nutrition consultation for perioperative nutritional plan

---

providers prescribing for each condition (**Box 11**). Additionally, because of changes in physiology, and especially renal function, older adults are at higher risk of experiencing adverse drug-drug and drug-person events. Some medications have been implicated as particularly high risk for adverse events and are listed by the American Geriatrics Society Beers Criteria as potentially inappropriate medications to be avoided.[25] Additionally, polypharmacy and certain medications increase the risk of postoperative delirium.[26] To minimize these adverse events, comprehensive medication management should include the following[2,25]:

1. Review and reconcile all medications: prescription, over-the-counter (especially pain and allergy/cold medicine), eye drops, topical, herbals, and other supplements
2. Confirm an indication for each medication
3. Check for drug-drug interactions
4. Adjust dosing appropriate for renal and liver function
5. Replace high-risk medications
6. Consider discontinuing nonessential medications
7. Specify if any medications should be stopped/started preoperatively
8. Avoid starting high-risk medications, especially:
   a. Benzodiazepines (except for treatment of alcohol withdrawal)
   b. Sedating antihistamines
   c. Meperidine for pain management

Treatment preferences are influenced by patients' expectations around outcomes, including anticipated functional status and need for care after a procedure (**Box 12**). In one study, most older adults with limited life expectancy stated they would undergo a low-burden treatment to restore current health, but would decline treatment if the outcome included survival with severe functional impairment or cognitive impairment (74.4% and 88.8%, respectively).[27] For these reasons, the ACS NSQIP-AGS guidelines recommend[2]

1. The patient have an advance directive and designated health care proxy or surrogate.
2. Discussion of the treatment goals and documentation of the patient's preferences and expectations.
3. Description of expected postoperative care and potential complications, including potential need for rehabilitation or nursing home care at discharge, if relevant.
4. Determination of patient's social support systems, which could impact discharge planning. Consider social work referral if social support is limited or inadequate.

Box 11
Medication

Assessment: medication reconciliation

Action: deprescribe, dose adjust, replace high-risk medications, document accurate medication list

---

Box 12
Patient counseling

Assessment: "Best Case/Worst Case" communication tool

Action: document health care proxy/surrogate, patient preferences/expectations, social support; social work referral

Data from Taylor LJ, Nabozny MJ, Steffens NM, et al. A framework to improve surgeon communication in high-stakes surgical decisions: best case/worst case. JAMA Surg 2017;152(6):531–8.

Patient decisions aids may facilitate the discussions. A 2014 Cochrane review found that when patients use decisions aides, they do improve knowledge of options, feel more informed and clear about what matters most to them, have more accurate expectations of possible benefits/harm, and participate more in decision making.[28] Shared decision making is crucial in reaching treatment decisions and in providing value-concordant care. However, communication, especially in the acute inpatient setting with seriously ill patients and their families, is challenging. The "Best Case/Worst Case" communication tool is one way for surgeons to engage older patients and their families in treatment decisions and to align treatment choices with patient preferences.[29] This strategy combines discussion with a hand-written graphic aid to illustrate choices between treatments to help engage patients and families. The provider uses stories to describe how patients might experience a range of possible outcomes in the best case, worst case, and most likely scenarios. These types of discussions allow patients and families to have a better understanding of their treatment choices and allow the provider to better understand the patients' preferences and treatment goals.

Studies have demonstrated the lack of reliable evidence underlying recommendations for preoperative testing and should be based on the patient's history and surgery planned (**Box 13**).[30] Unnecessary testing should be avoided because of the burden to the patient, cost to the health system, and lack of evidence showing benefit. For older adults, routine preoperative screening tests are not recommended with the exception of hemoglobulin, renal function (bun/cr), and serum albumin because they inform other components of the preoperative evaluation and also allow appropriate dosing of medications that are administered during and after the procedure. Additional testing should be performed based on the patient characteristics and planned procedure (**Table 1**).

SUMMARY

Older adults are at higher risk for postoperative complications because of increased rates of multimorbidity, polypharmacy, functional changes, and cognitive impairment. Appropriate preoperative evaluation assesses operative and postoperative risk factors and identifies areas to mitigate risk and also to clarify treatment expectations

---

Box 13
Preoperative testing

Assessment: careful history and review of planned procedure

Action: renal function, hemoglobulin, serum albumin; additional testing based on patient history and planned procedure

---

Table 1 Indications for preoperative testing	
Test	**Indication**
White blood cell count	Myeloproliferative disease or at high risk for leukopenia from drugs or other known disease
Platelet count	High likelihood of thrombocytopenia or thrombocytosis
Coagulation tests (PT/INR/PTT)	History of bleeding disorders, on medications affecting coagulation, on warfarin, or on hemodialysis Surgeries associated with bleeding or high risk of complications from bleeding, such as arterial reconstruction, cardiac surgery, cancer operations, spine procedures Malnutrition, malabsorption, or liver disease
Electrolytes (Na, K, Cl, CO_2)	Baseline renal insufficiency, congestive heart failure Taking diuretics, digoxin, angiotensin-converting enzyme inhibitors, or other medications that increase likelihood of abnormal results
Serum glucose	Known or suspected diabetes, or obesity
Urinalysis	Suspected urinary tract infection, known diabetes, or undergoing urogenital surgery
CXR	Acute cardiopulmonary disease (including smoking, asthma, and COPD) >70 y old with history of stable chronic cardiopulmonary disease without recent CXR in past 6 mo Possible ICU stay, obtain for baseline CXR Undergoing major surgery
Electrocardiogram	Undergoing intermediate-risk or vascular surgery Known ischemic heart disease, previous myocardial infarction, cardiac arrhythmias, peripheral vascular disease, cerebrovascular diseases, compensated or prior heart failure, diabetes, renal insufficiency, or respiratory disease
Pulmonary function tests	Undergoing lung resection Poorly characterized dyspnea or exercise intolerance with diagnostic uncertainty between cardiac or pulmonary limitation vs simple deconditioning Obstructive lung disease with questionable preoperative optimization
Noninvasive stress testing	>3 clinical risk factors and poor functional capacity (<4 METs) undergoing vascular surgery >1 clinical risk factor and poor functional capacity (<4 METs) undergoing intermediate risk or vascular surgery, if it changes management

Abbreviations: CXR, chest radiograph; ICU, intensive care unit; INR, international normalized ratio; PT, prothrombin time; PTT, partial thromboplastin time.

From Chow WB, Rosenthal RA, Merkow RP, et al. Optimal preoperative assessment of the geriatric surgical patient: a best practices guideline from the American College of Surgeons National Surgical Quality Improvement Program and the American Geriatrics Society. J Am Coll Surg 2012;215(4):453–66; with permission.

and outcomes. The optimal preoperative evaluation for older adults addresses medical conditions and other areas pertinent to the care of older adults including assessments of cognition, capacity, delirium risk, function, frailty, nutrition, medications, and treatment preferences (**Box 14**).

Box 14
Summary of preoperative assessment domains for older adults

Cognition/capacity

Assessment: Mini-Cog,[4] Patient Health Questionnaire-2,[5] capacity assessment

Action: educate on associated risks, establish health care proxy, document capacity

Alcohol/substance screening

Assessment: CAGE[7]

Action: multivitamin with folate, thiamine; close monitoring for signs of withdrawal

Delirium risk

Assessment: assess risk factors

Action: implement management plan to mitigate modifiable risk factor, including education of patients and families.

Cardiac

Assessment: American College of Cardiology and American Heart Association algorithm[10]

Action: cardiac testing and optimization based on risk assessment

Pulmonary

Assessment: history of pulmonary risk factors

Action: mitigate risk factors, as able; smoking cessation

Function/falls

Assessment: Activities of daily living,[17] hearing/vision screen, falls history, Timed Up and Go Test[18]

Action: physical therapy, assistive supportive

Frailty

Assessment: Fried Frailty Index[19]

Action: exercise program, nutritional support, "prehab"

Nutrition

Assessment options: serum albumin, body mass index

Action: nutrition consultation for perioperative nutritional plan

Medication

Assessment: medication reconciliation

Action: deprescribe, dose adjust, replace high-risk medications, document accurate medication list

Patient counseling

Assessment: "Best Case/Worst Case"[29]

Action: document health care proxy/surrogate, patient preferences/expectations, social support; social work referral

Preoperative testing

Assessment: careful history and review of planned procedure

Action: renal function, hemoglobulin, serum albumin; additional testing based on patient history and planned procedure

Data from Refs.[4,5,7,10,17–19,29]

REFERENCES

1. C W. The older population: 2010. Washington, DC: U.S. Census Bureau; 2011.
2. Chow WB, Rosenthal RA, Merkow RP, et al. Optimal preoperative assessment of the geriatric surgical patient: a best practices guideline from the American College of Surgeons National Surgical Quality Improvement Program and the American Geriatrics Society. J Am Coll Surg 2012;215(4):453–66.
3. American Geriatrics Society Expert Panel on Postoperative Delirium in Older Adults. American Geriatrics Society abstracted clinical practice guideline for postoperative delirium in older adults. J Am Geriatr Soc 2015;63(1):142–50.
4. Borson S, Scanlan J, Chen P, et al. The mini-cog as a screen for dementia: validation in a population-based sample. J Am Geriatr Soc 2003;51(10):1451–4.
5. Li C, Friedman B, Conwell Y, et al. Validity of the patient health questionnaire 2 (PHQ-2) in identifying major depression in older people. J Am Geriatr Soc 2007;55:596–602.
6. Appelbaum P. Clinical practice. Assessment of patients' competence to consent to treatment. N Engl J Med 2007;357(18):1834–40.
7. Hinkin C, Castellon S, Dickson-Fuhrman E, et al. Screening for drug and alcohol abuse among older adults using a modified version of the CAGE. Am J Addict 2001;10(4):319–26.
8. Inouye S. Current concepts. Delirium in older persons. N Engl J Med 2006;354: 1157–65.
9. Mohanty S, Rosenthal RA, Russell MM, et al. Optimal perioperative management of the geriatric patient: a best practices guideline from the American College of Surgeons NSQIP and the American Geriatrics Society. J Am Coll Surg 2016; 222(5):930–47.
10. Fleisher LA, Fleischmann KE, Auerbach AD, et al. 2014 ACC/AHA guideline on perioperative cardiovascular evaluation and management of patients undergoing noncardiac surgery: a report of the American College of Cardiology/American Heart Association Task Force on practice guidelines. J Am Coll Cardiol 2014; 64(22):e77–137.
11. Gleason LJ, Friedman SM. Preoperative management of anticoagulation and antiplatelet agents. Clin Geriatr Med 2014;30(2):219–27.
12. Doherty JU, Gluckman TJ, Hucker WJ, et al. 2017 ACC expert consensus decision pathway for periprocedural management of anticoagulation in patients with nonvalvular atrial fibrillation: a report of the American College of Cardiology Clinical Expert Consensus Document Task Force. J Am Coll Cardiol 2017;69(7): 871–98.
13. Fernandez-Bustamante A, Frendl G, Sprung J, et al. Postoperative pulmonary complications, early mortality, and hospital stay following noncardiothoracic surgery: a multicenter study by the perioperative research network investigators. JAMA Surg 2017;152(2):157–66.
14. Smetana G. Preoperative pulmonary assessment of the older adult. Clin Geriatr Med 2003;19(1):35–55.
15. Smetana G, Lawrence V, Cornell J. Preoperative pulmonary risk stratification for noncardiothoracic surgery: systematic review for the American College of Physicians. Ann Intern Med 2006;144(8):581–95.
16. Min L, Hall K, Finlayson E, et al. Estimating risk of postsurgical general and geriatric complications using the VESPA preoperative tool. JAMA Surg 2017;152(12): 1126–33.

17. Katz S, Downs T, Cash H, et al. Progress in development of the index of AD. Gerontologist 1970;10:20–30.

18. Podsiadlo D, Richardson S. The timed "Up & Go": a test of basic functional mobility for frail elderly persons. J Am Geriatr Soc 1991;39:142–8.

19. Makary MA, Segev DL, Pronovost PJ, et al. Frailty as a predictor of surgical outcomes in older patients. J Am Coll Surg 2010;210(6):901–8.

20. Adams P, Ghanem T, Stachler R, et al. Frailty as a predictor of morbidity and mortality in inpatient head and neck surgery. JAMA Otolaryngol Head Neck Surg 2013;139(8):783–9.

21. Carli F, Scheede-Bergdahl C. Prehabilitation to enhance perioperative care. Anesthesiol Clin 2015;33(1):17–33.

22. Liu CK, Fielding RA. Exercise as an intervention for frailty. Clin Geriatr Med 2011; 27(1):101–10.

23. Curtis LJ, Bernier P, Jeejeebhoy K, et al. Costs of hospital malnutrition. Clin Nutr 2017;36(5):1391–6.

24. Baldwin C, Weekes CE. Dietary advice with or without oral nutritional supplements for disease-related malnutrition in adults. Cochrane Database Syst Rev 2011;(9):CD002008.

25. By the American Geriatrics Society Beers Criteria Update Expert Panel. American Geriatrics Society 2015 updated beers criteria for potentially inappropriate medication use in older adults. J Am Geriatr Soc 2015;63(11):2227–46.

26. Jeong YM, Lee E, Kim KI, et al. Association of pre-operative medication use with post-operative delirium in surgical oncology patients receiving comprehensive geriatric assessment. BMC Geriatr 2016;16:134.

27. Fried T, Bradley E, Towle V, et al. Understanding the treatment preferences of seriously ill patients. N Engl J Med 2002;346(14):1061–6.

28. Stacey D, Legare F, Col NF, et al. Decision aids for people facing health treatment or screening decisions. Cochrane Database Syst Rev 2014;(1):CD001431.

29. Taylor LJ, Nabozny MJ, Steffens NM, et al. A framework to improve surgeon communication in high-stakes surgical decisions: best case/worst case. JAMA Surg 2017;152(6):531–8.

30. Martin S, Cifu A. Routine preoperative laboratory tests for elective surgery. JAMA 2007;318(6):567–8.

The Emerging Field of Geriatric Otolaryngology

David Eibling, MD[a],*, Karen Kost, MD[b]

KEYWORDS

- Geriatric Otolaryngology • Subspecialty education • American Geriatric Society
- Geriatrics for Specialists Initiatives • Dennis Jahnigen grants
- American Society of Geriatric Otolaryngology

KEY POINTS

- Current and anticipated dramatic increases in the number of older adults seeking care for disorders of the head and neck will require that more otolaryngologists have the skills to manage these patients.
- Advances in knowledge and technology drive sub specialization in all specialties, including Otolaryngology-Head and Neck Surgery, but for a variety of reasons a new distinct sub-specialty of geriatric otolaryngology is unlikely to be formed.
- The optimal solution to the challenge presented by the new needs is increased education of otolaryngologists in gerontology and specifically geriatric otolaryngology.

INTRODUCTION

The readers of this issue of the *Otolaryngologic Clinics of North America* need no reminder that many of the complaints that drive older adults to seek treatment originate in the anatomic region of the head and neck. It has been estimated that roughly one-third of all visits for specific complaints relate to the anatomic and physiologic regions that have been managed by practitioners of the ear, nose, and throat (ENT).

HISTORY OF OTOLARYNGOLOGY

A review of the history of the specialty of Otolaryngology-Head and Neck Surgery will help frame the story of Geriatric Otolaryngology. Otolaryngology as a specialty has existed for more than a century, and 2 of the larger otolaryngologic professional organizations have recently celebrated 100 years since their formation. The American

Disclosure: The authors have nothing to disclose.
[a] Department of Otolaryngology-HNS, University of Pittsburgh School of Medicine, 200 Lothrop Street, Pittsburgh, PA 15213, USA; [b] Department of Otolaryngology-HNS, McGill University School of Medicine, 1001 Decarie Boulevard, Montreal, Québec H4A 3J1, Canada
* Corresponding author.
E-mail address: eiblingde@upmc.edu

Board of Otolaryngology is one of the oldest boards, predated only by the American Board of Ophthalmology. The specialty arose from recognition by practitioners that specific knowledge, skills, and instrumentation were required to manage these disorders. Early otolaryngologists practiced as "eye, ear, nose, and throat surgeons," and the parent organization did not separate into respective Ophthalmology and Otolaryngology academies until the 1970s. Older patients still often assume that their otolaryngologists practice "EENT." Early otolaryngologists possessed the skills to visualize, diagnose, and treat diseases of the ear. In the preantibiotic era, most interventions were to manage infections. For example, today it is difficult to imagine the significance of a common disease, otitis media, at the time. Approximately 75% of children will suffer at least one episode of otitis media. Without effective treatment, the infection in some affected children progressed to coalescent mastoiditis (essentially osteomyelitis of the skull base) and then often complications such as septic thrombosis of draining veins, intracranial abscesses, or meningitis. Physicians trained in otolaryngology routinely opened infected mastoids using a hammer, chisels, and gouges to drain the infection, thereby saving the child's life. Many of these children were left with residual tympanic membrane perforations and hearing loss. Eye and ear hospitals sprung up in major cities to enable these and other surgical procedures, chiefly for management of infection. The father of one of the authors (D.E.) related visiting a children's ward as a child himself in the late 1920s and being struck by the number of children (he recalled there were at least a dozen) wearing white mastoid dressings. It is likely that many of the readers of this article have in their practices patients in their 9th and 10th decades of life who underwent "simple" mastoidectomies in childhood as a life-saving maneuver in the preantibiotic era.

Over the intervening years, multiple other interventions for management of diseases of the ear, nose, and throat became standard within the specialty, including the addition of surgery for head and neck cancer approximately 50 years ago, With the widespread employment of antibiotics, the practice of otolaryngology shifted dramatically, and most of the Eye and Ear Hospitals have closed and their functions assimilated into children's hospitals as well as general hospitals. The paradigm of a recognized need driving the development of a specialty, or subspecialty, continues to this day as will be outlined in next.

HISTORY OF PEDIATRIC OTOLARYNGOLOGY

Reviewing the development of the subspecialty of pediatric otolaryngology can provide a frame for the discussion of the development of geriatric otolaryngology in this article.

A half century ago, at about the time today's older otolaryngologists were beginning their active practice, insightful practitioners of the specialty recognized that some children presented unique clinical and therapeutic challenges, which extended beyond the knowledge and skills of many practicing in the specialty. These leaders embarked on a legendary quest to develop new techniques to evaluate and manage these children. In order to focus their activities, they established new departments or divisions within the pediatric hospitals already in existence. Over the intervening years, new societies focusing on the otolaryngologic diseases of children were formed to facilitate information sharing. Specialized training programs were established throughout the world, so that subspecialists in pediatric otolaryngology are found in all academic departments and practice in all children's hospitals. Sophisticated scientific investigations within these departments have yielded new knowledge regarding the care of children with diseases of the ears, nose, and throat. The subspecialty of pediatric otolaryngology is now firmly established, and today's practitioners could not imagine an academic department without trained pediatric otolaryngologists. These subspecialists have assumed the responsibility of training not only pediatric-otolaryngology subspecialists but also general otolaryngologists in the basic knowledge and skills necessary to manage children with otolaryngologic disorders. Mirroring the remarkable advances elsewhere across the science and practice of medicine, the subspecialty has introduced dramatic innovations, such as the development of EXIT (Ex Utero Intrapartum Treatment) procedures to correct otherwise fatal congenital airway disorders, the widespread recognition and knowledge of the management of developmental abnormalities, as well as the widespread utilization of cochlear implantation for children with congenital deafness. Investigations in many institutions have yielded high-level evidence that provides the foundation for the development of clinical practice guidelines that assist in point-of-care decision-making for the management of common childhood aliments, such as chronic tonsillitis, sleep-disordered breathing, and chronic middle ear effusions. It seems axiomatic that these and other advances are a direct result of the recognition by early leaders in the subspecialty that children were not just "little adults" and that their distinct physiology required a unique approach by specialized practitioners, investigators, and teachers.

GERIATRIC OTOLARYNGOLOGY

A quarter of a century later, insightful otolaryngologists reached the same conclusion regarding the care of the elderly, recognizing the rapid increase in the numbers of geriatric patients and that they are more than just "older adults." However, for several reasons, the dramatic changes witnessed in pediatric otolaryngology have not occurred, resulting in evolutionary change rather than the dramatic changes that accompanied the development of pediatric otolaryngology.

With the exception of the pediatric subspecialists, all otolaryngologists manage older adults on a daily basis. Recognition of the profound differences in the disease processes, personal goals, and therapeutic choices of elderly patients, when compared with younger individuals, frequently eludes practitioners. Moreover, until recently there has been relatively little research focused on the unique physiology and therapeutic responses of elderly patients. The formation of a separate subspecialty of geriatric otolaryngology is unlikely because most otolaryngologists manage diseases and disorders in older adults. Alternatively, efforts should be channeled into a strategy focused on (i) supporting research to define the characteristics of otolaryngologic disease in older adults, (ii) the education of both general and subspecialty otolaryngologists in basic gerontology, and specialty-specific management of their geriatric patients.

HISTORY OF GERIATRIC OTOLARYNGOLOGY

The early history of geriatric otolaryngology is actually quite recent. Some 30 years ago, Jerome (Jerry) Goldstein, at the time the executive vice president of what is now the American Academy of Otolaryngology-Head and Neck Surgery (AAO-HNS), recognized the pressing need to disseminate age-specific geriatric knowledge and skills to practicing otolaryngologists. To this end, he organized a symposium focused on Geriatric Otolaryngology, held in Washington DC in the mid 1980s. This symposium is widely considered to constitute the first educational initiative focused on teaching the principles of geriatrics as they pertain to the specialty of otolaryngology and resulted in the first book specifically addressing the principles of geriatric otolaryngology.[1]

Despite this auspicious beginning, little occurred within the specialty of otolaryngology over the next decade. Within the geriatric community, however, there was a hum of activity. They recognized the demographic shifts that were occurring, a decade before most of the rest of the house of medicine. Indeed, they anticipated the inadequacy of resources available to manage the approaching enormous numbers of aging "baby boomers" about to hit, and overwhelm, the US health care system. Leaders within the American Geriatric Society (AGS), led by Dennis Jahnigen, understood that there would never be sufficient numbers of trained geriatricians to meet the needs of this "tsunami" of geriatric patients. Not only were the large numbers of "boomers" going to transition to "older adults" over a relatively short period, but also they were likely to expect much more from the health care system in order to sustain a high quality of life. They would not be content to sit in rockers, but would want to exercise, hear, swallow, and communicate at a high level, and in doing so inevitably use health care resources to a previously unanticipated degree. The Institute of Medicine initially predicted this challenge in 1978 and then published another report in 2008 in which the authors stated in the opening summary on page 1, *"While this population surge has been foreseen for decades, little has been done to prepare the health care workforce for its arrival. . . . . Unless action is taken immediately, the health care workforce will lack the capacity (in both size and ability) to meet the needs of older patients in the future."*[2]

Anticipating this challenge long before the Institute of Medicine reports, and recognizing that they could not meet the needs of future geriatric patients unaided, the AGS adopted a strategy of educating specialists in the principles of geriatrics. In 1994, with the collaboration and generous funding from the John A. Hartford foundation, the AGS launched a multipronged approach, the Geriatrics for Specialists Initiative (GSI), outlined in a recent article in the *Journal of the American Geriatric Society*.[3]

THE AMERICAN GERIATRICS FOR SPECIALISTS INITIATIVE

The GSI was established by the AGS in 1994 to spearhead efforts to support research into diseases of the elderly as well as education of specialists in basic gerontology. Through this initiative, the AGS established collaborative workgroups with 11 other medical and surgical specialties, including the AAO-HNS. The multifaceted approach stimulated joint development of educational programs initially focused on teaching basic geriatric principles to otolaryngology residents. The AGS funded several educational grants to otolaryngology departments to create enduring instruction materials. Other efforts focused on promoting specialty-specific geriatric research. Supported by funding from the John A. Hartford Foundation, career development grants were awarded to young investigators who would focus their research activities on disorders of the elderly within their respective specialty. Several of these "Dennis Jahnigen" grants (named for the early leader of the AGS GSI program) supported a research portfolio that addressed the unique challenges older adults present when seeking care for otolaryngologic diseases. Several otolaryngologist-investigators are continuing to work on projects that sprang from these grants, assuming leadership roles within the specialty in promulgating the principles of geriatric otolaryngology. By any measure, the GSI has been successful in moving the otolaryngology community forward toward a more focused attention on geriatric otolaryngology.

ORGANIZED OTOLARYNGOLOGY

The AAO-HNS established a geriatric committee to promote the effective involvement of the national organization and its members in geriatric otolaryngology. In retrospect, it seems likely that this effort was at least in part due to the initiative of the AGS GSI. This committee has been active in generating enduring text material, both online and in print format to educate otolaryngologists in basic geriatric principles.[4]

Recognizing the need for geriatric competencies, the leadership of the American Board of Otolaryngology initiated a program to assure that board-certified otolaryngologists possess basic knowledge of general and specialty-specific geriatric topics. This effort has occurred in synchrony with other specialties represented by the American Board of Medical Specialties. Current competencies cross surgical specialties, although specialty-specific competencies are being developed. Major topics include frailty, cognitive change, surgical decision making, and end-of-life decision making.

THE AMERICAN SOCIETY OF GERIATRIC OTOLARYNGOLOGY

In the mid-2000s, nearly 2 decades after the Cherry Blossom symposium he had organized, Jerry Goldstein recognized that further progress would require the establishment of a subspecialty society. Hence, in collaboration with George Gates, he conceptualized and established the American Society of Geriatric Otolaryngology (ASGO) in 2006. Jerry served as its first president, and George as its treasurer. The authors of this article served as the first secretary (D.E.) and program chair (K.K.) of the fledgling organization. The society has held annual meetings every year since 2007, initially just before the Combined Otolaryngology Spring Meetings and more recently during the Triological Society Combined Winter Meetings. The society is "inclusive" in that members do not need to be of any specific specialty, the only requirement being that they be practitioners with an interest in geriatric otolaryngology. The society provides associate membership to allied professionals such as audiologists, as well as physical and speech therapists. Reasonable dues cover registration to the annual meeting. ASGO is a "paperless" society, and information is disseminated via its Web site, www.geriatricotolaryngology.org. Readers of this article are encouraged to access the site for more information and to consider joining the organization.

Topics addressed at the annual meeting include dysphagia, balance disorders, end-of-life discussions, and frailty, particularly as it relates to surgical decision making. More recently, investigations into the association between cognitive decline and central hearing loss have led to several presentations on the topic. Through the efforts of the ASGO leadership, many of geriatric topics have been incorporated into presentations at general otolaryngologic meetings, both regional and national. ASGO members have prepared and presented several instruction courses and mini seminars sponsored by the geriatric committee of the AAO-HNS, presented at the annual meeting. In 2014, ASGO members delivered presentations on sleep disorders in the elderly, and frailty at a Triological Plenary session, with more presentations in several formats currently under development.

Members of the society are well represented on the AAO-HNS geriatric committee as well as many other multispecialty geriatric task forces. Members of the society have taken an active role in committee and guideline development activities of the AAO-HNS and the Canadian Society of Otolaryngology (CSO) as well as participated in several advocacy efforts to enhance otolaryngologic care delivery to the elderly of our nations.

Despite its small size and "youthful" existence of barely a decade, ASGO is continuing to impact the development of a geriatric focus within the specialty of otolaryngology.

CHALLENGES FACING GERIATRIC OTOLARYNGOLOGY

Those that manage geriatric patients are well aware of the challenges in disseminating information and inducing specialists to devote the time and energy required to treat older adults. Otolaryngology is not exempt from these challenges. Not only are care decisions often much more difficult, but also the intrinsic auditory and cognitive abilities of many patients impair doctor-patient communication. Moreover, issues with social support and caregiver availability (not to mention occasional disagreements) often require the investment of far more time than is given in the typical adult otolaryngology encounter. In a high-volume otolaryngology outpatient practice, office encounters may be limited to 15 to 20 minutes each. Managing geriatric patients with multiple comorbidities simply requires more time than is typically allotted.

Another challenge is the fact that otolaryngologists are, at heart, procedure driven. Much of the treatment they dispense is through procedures, in either the outpatient office or the operating room. As most geriatric patients do not require procedural intervention, there is less interest in learning geriatric skills within the specialty. Moreover, the specialty emphasis on reimbursement for procedures represents a significant deterrent for many physicians. Finally, the disparate reimbursement by payers for "cognitive work" (well known to geriatricians) further reduces the interest in developing an emphasis on managing the geriatric otolaryngologic patients within the specialty.

THE FUTURE

Demographic changes will inevitably increase the number of older patients seeking otolaryngologic care. As has been demonstrated by the actions of the AGS, and now emulated by the AAO-HNS, the ABO, the CSO, and ASGO, education of otolaryngologists in basic geriatric principles as well as management of otolaryngologic-specific disorders is the optimal strategy. The readers of this article are encouraged to seek opportunities in which they can participate in educational endeavors within their academic institutions and local communities.

REFERENCES

1. Goldstein JR, editor. Geriatric otolaryngology. Philidelphia: Dekker; 1988.
2. Institute of Medicine. Retooling for an aging America: building the health care workforce. Washington, DC: The National Academies Press; 2008. https://doi.org/10.17226/12089.
3. Lee AG, Burton JA, Lundebjerg NE. The geriatrics-for-specialists initiative: an eleven specialty collaboration to improve the care of older adults. J Am Geriatr Soc 2017;65(10):2140–5.
4. Sataloff RT, Johns MM, Kost KM. Geriatric otolaryngology. New York: Thieme; 2015. ISBN9781626239777.

Moving?

Make sure your subscription moves with you!

To notify us of your new address, find your **Clinics Account Number** (located on your mailing label above your name), and contact customer service at:

Email: journalscustomerservice-usa@elsevier.com

800-654-2452 (subscribers in the U.S. & Canada)
314-447-8871 (subscribers outside of the U.S. & Canada)

Fax number: 314-447-8029

Elsevier Health Sciences Division
Subscription Customer Service
3251 Riverport Lane
Maryland Heights, MO 63043

*To ensure uninterrupted delivery of your subscription, please notify us at least 4 weeks in advance of move.